GP ST: Stage 2
Practice Questions

PasTest

to your success

GP ST: Stage 2
Practice Questions

**Edited by Sean Coughlin,
MBChB FRCGP MMedSc**

General Practitioner

Lancashire

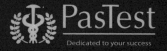

PasTest
Dedicated to your success

© 2007 PASTEST LTD
Egerton Court
Parkgate Estate
Knutsford
Cheshire
WA16 8DX

Telephone: 01565 752000

First Published 2007

ISBN: 1905 635 400

978 1905 635 405

A catalogue record for this book is available from the British Library.

The information contained within this book was obtained by the author from reliable sources. However, while every effort has been made to ensure its accuracy, no responsibility for loss, damage or injury occasioned to any person acting or refraining from action as a result of information contained herein can be accepted by the publishers or author.

PasTest Revision Books and Intensive Courses

PasTest has been established in the field of postgraduate medical education since 1972, providing revision books and intensive study courses for doctors preparing for their professional examinations.

Books and courses are available for the following specialties:
MRCGP, MRCP Parts 1 and 2, MRCPCH Parts 1 and 2, MRCPsych, MRCS, MRCOG Parts 1 and 2, DRCOG, DCH, FRCA, PLAB Parts 1 and 2.

For further details contact:

PasTest, Freepost, Knutsford, Cheshire WA16 7BR

Tel: 01565 752000 Fax: 01565 650264

www.pastest.co.uk enquiries@pastest.co.uk

Text prepared by Carnegie Book Production, Lancaster

Printed and bound by Page Bros, Norwich, UK

CONTENTS

CONTRIBUTORS

EDITOR

Sean Coughlin, MB ChB, FRCGP, MMedSc
General Practitioner
Lancashire

CONTRIBUTORS

Paul Anderson, BSc (Hons), MB ChB (Hons), FRCS(Urol)
Consultant Urological Surgeon
Dudley

Angela Bennett, MB BChir
GP Registrar
York Street Medical Practice
Cambridge

Julia Dancy, MB ChB, MRCP (UK), DCH, DTM&H
GP Registrar
Croydon VTS
London Deanery

Arwa Eskander, MB ChB (Sheffield)
Foundation Year 2 Respiratory Medicine
University Hospital of North Staffordshire

Brandon John, MB ChB (Sheffield)
Foundation Year 2 Paediatrics
Stafford General Hospital
Stafford

Stephanie-Jayne Jones, BClin Sci, MB ChB, MRCP, MRCGP,
DipPharmMed
Sessional General Practitioner/Drug Safety Physician
Cheshire

Priya Joshi, MB ChB, MRCGP
Sessional General Practitioner
Cambridge

Louise Newson, BSc(Hons), MB ChB (Hons), MRCP MRCGP
General Practitioner
Solihull
West Midlands

Laura Weidner, MB ChB (UK)
Foundation Year 2 Doctor
Accident and Emergency
Walsall Hospitals NHS Trust
Walsall

INTRODUCTION

There is a nationally agreed and quality assured process of appointment to general practitioner (GP) specialty training, coordinated by the National Recruitment Office. Full details of the process can be found on the Office's website (www.gprecruitment.org.uk).

Currently, there are four stages in the process:

- Stage 1 (long-list) consists of filling an application form, providing personal and professional details. If a candidate's details meet the essential eligibility criteria, the application is accepted.

- Stage 2 (short-list) is an assessment conducted under exam conditions. The rest of this book is about this stage, and provides advice and material to help candidates prepare for and successfully negotiate the assessment.

- Stage 3 (selection) consists of an assessment at a selection centre. An invitation to attend will be sent to those candidates achieving a high enough score in Stage 2. At the selection centre, candidates are assessed in a variety of tasks, such as a patient simulation exercise and group exercise.

  Stages 1–3 of the assessment process are blue-printed against the national person specification (www.gprecruitment.org.uk) which is itself based on Good Medical Practice. (www.gmc-uk.org/guidance/good_medical_practice/index.asp).

- Stage 4 (allocation and offer) follows for successful candidates. The candidates who scored the highest in Stage 3 and the relevant parts of Stage 2 are most likely to be offered the programmes of their choice. If a deanery cannot offer a post to a suitable candidate, the candidate can be offered a post at another deanery via the national clearing process of the National Recruitment Office.

Clinical Problem Solving Questions

INTRODUCTION TO CLINICAL PROBLEM SOLVING QUESTIONS

The purpose of GP training is to provide the trainee with the necessary competences to practise independently as a general practitioner (www.rcgp-curriculum.org.uk), not to pump knowledge into an individual. However, a candidate is expected, after 5–6 years as a medical student and 2 years as a foundation doctor, to have a reasonable level of knowledge and to be able to apply it to clinical situations. This is what the first part of Stage 2 assesses.

The assessment consists of a 90-minute question paper. The questions are in the form of clinical scenarios that require candidates to exercise judgement and problem solving skills to determine the appropriate diagnosis and management of patients. The level of difficulty of the questions will be such that a year 2 foundation programme doctor could reasonably be expected to answer. Thus, none of the questions require specific knowledge about general practice.

The questions are evenly distributed across specific topic areas:

- Cardiovascular
- Dermatology/ENT/eye
- Endocrinology/metabolic
- Gastroenterology/nutrition
- Infectious disease/haematology/immunology/genetics
- Musculoskeletal
- Paediatrics
- Pharmacology/therapeutics
- Psychiatry/neurology
- Reproductive (male and female)
- Renal/urology
- Respiratory

Questions will relate to:

- Disease factors

- Making a diagnosis

- Investigations

- Management

- Prescribing

- Emergency care

The questions may appear in a variety of formats but two formats are commonly used, Extending Matching Questions and Single Best Answer Questions. In both formats, candidates have to choose the most likely of the given possible responses to a question, according to their clinical judgement. Unless otherwise stated, only one answer is required. It will often be an answer that could be found in a nationally approved guideline or the *British National Formulary*. Other answers may be plausible, but one will clearly be the most appropriate.

A sample Extending Matching Question and Single Best Answer Question are given below.

EXTENDED MATCHING QUESTION

In Extending Matching Questions, a number of scenarios relating to a 'theme' are matched to the most appropriate choice from a list of options.

Example

THEME: FEBRILE CHILDREN

A Chickenpox

B Erythema infectiosum

C Hand, foot and mouth disease

D Herpangina

E Herpes simplex

F Rubella

G Scarlet fever

H Vincent angina

For each clinical scenario given below, select the single most likely diagnosis from the list above. Each option may be selected once, more than once or not at all.

☐ 1   A 4-year-old boy is pyrexial and has a sore throat and an erythematous rash that spares the area around the mouth. The tongue is red with prominent papillae.

☐ 2   A 5-year-old girl has been unwell for 2 days. She now has oedematous erythematous plaques on the cheeks.

☐ 3   A 3-year-old girl has a sore mouth with diffuse ulceration. She is dripping saliva and there are vesicles around her mouth.

☐ 4   A 2-year-old boy develops crops of vesicles on an erythematous base on the head, body and arms. The crops appear in different stages. There are ulcers in the mouth.

Answers

1   **G**   Scarlet fever

2   **B**   Erythema infectiosum

3   **E**   Herpes simplex

4   **A**   Chickenpox

SINGLE BEST ANSWER QUESTION

Single Best Answer Questions consist of a statement followed by a number of items, *one* of which is correct.

Example

1   **A 34-year-old woman returns 7 days after receiving chloramphenicol eye drops for apparent conjunctivitis. Her eyes feel gritty and water. There is diffuse injection of the sclera.**

        Select the single most likely diagnosis from the list below.

☐ **A**   Bacterial conjunctivitis
☐ **B**   Episcleritis
☐ **C**   Iritis
☐ **D**   Keratitis
☐ **E**   Viral conjunctivitis

Answer E   Viral conjunctivitis

Occasionally, more than one answer may be required (Multiple Best Answer Question) so it is important to read each question carefully. Beside clinical scenarios, results of investigations may also be presented. Photographs or electrocardiograms may also be included.

Each correct answer is awarded one mark and the total score equals the number of correct answers. The score required to proceed to Stage 3 varies from year to year and depends on many factors, not least of which is how hard the paper is thought to be. This implies that a few hard questions can be expected. The purpose of the test is to distinguish between high and low achieving candidates and if all the questions are easy that task will be much more difficult. A few of the examples in this book are in the difficult category for the same reason.

There is no negative marking in this test (ie the loss of a mark when an incorrect answer is given). This removes the 'fear factor'. Candidates should pace themselves carefully and not run out of time. Where an answer is not known an intelligent guess should be made. No questions should be left unanswered as this may artificially lower the mark.

A lot of thought is given to the wording of the questions to try to make them as unambiguous as possible. However, it is important that candidates understand the meaning of certain conventional terms which frequently appear in the paper. These will be provided with the paper and can be found on the National Recruitment Office website. They are reproduced below and may appear in some of the questions in this book.

- *Pathognomic, diagnostic, characteristic* and *in the vast majority* imply that a feature would occur in at least 90% of cases.

- *Typically, frequently, significantly, commonly* and *in a substantial majority* imply that a feature would occur in at least 60% of cases.

- *In the majority* implies that a feature occurs in greater than 50% of cases.

- *In the minority* implies that a feature occurs in less than 50% of cases.

- *Low chance* and *in a substantial minority* imply that a feature may occur in up to 30% of cases.

- *Has been shown, recognised* and *reported* all refer to evidence that can be found in authoritative medical texts. None of these terms make any implication about the frequency with which the feature occurs.

Candidates who do not already do so should start reading thoroughly. Review articles and editorials in major journals are useful. Weaknesses in the minor specialties can be covered by reading books such as the *ABC of Dermatology* and the *ABC of Eyes* (both published by BMJ Publishing Group). It is useful to be aware of the main conclusions presented in the different sections of *Clinical Evidence* (BMJ Publishing Group; www.clinicalevidence. com). A good working knowledge of the *British National Formulary* will be invaluable. Lastly, there is no substitute for seeing plenty of patients and reflecting on the diagnostic and management issues presented, and the effect of the illness on a patient's life.

Chapter 1
Cardiovascular

QUESTIONS

THEME: CHEST PAIN

Options

A Coronary artery spasm
B Dissection of thoracic aorta
C Gastro-oesophageal reflux disease
D Mesothelioma
E Metastatic lung deposits
F Oesophageal spasm
G Pericarditis
H Pneumonia
I Pneumothorax
J Pulmonary embolism
K Tietze disease
L Unstable angina

From each of the case scenarios given below, select the single most appropriate diagnosis from the above list of options. Each option may be used once, more than once or not at all.

☐ **1.1** **A 25-year-old man has central chest pain, tachycardia and sweating. He has taken cocaine.**

☐ **1.2** **A 63-year-old male smoker has long-term hypertension. He has severe chest pain radiating to his back.**

☐ **1.3** **A 37-year-old woman has severe left-sided pain, which is worse on inspiration. She has antiphospholipid syndrome and a swollen left ankle.**

☐ **1.4**   A 42-year-old man has central chest pain. Movement exacerbates the pain and the anterior chest wall is tender.

☐ **1.5**   A 67-year-old male industrial worker has left-sided chest pain and long-term pleural plaques.

☐ **1.6**   An obese 42-year-old woman has central chest pain going through to her back, and this is worse in bed.

THEME: BASIC LIFE SUPPORT MANAGEMENT

Options

A   Check airway

B   Check pulse

C   Continue cardiopulmonary resuscitation (CPR) until exhausted

D   Give rescue breaths

E   Leave patient

F   No action

G   Place in recovery position

H   Start chest compressions

For each of the patients below, choose the single most appropriate treatment from the list of options above. Each option may be used once, more than once or not at all.

☐ **1.7** A 6-year-old has stopped breathing in the supermarket. You have given mouth-to-mouth ventilation. What do you do next?

☐ **1.8** A 73-year-old male visitor collapses in the hospital shop. You are the only other person in the shop. You open his airway and find he is not breathing.

☐ **1.9** A 43-year-old man collapses in the street. After you open his airway he starts groaning.

☐ **1.10** You rescue a 17-year-old boy from under the water in a canal. He is in cardiac arrest. You perform cardiopulmonary resuscitation alone for 1 minute and stop to assess your next action. The patient is unresponsive and cold.

☐ **1.11** There has been a bomb blast at a London underground train station and the man in the seat next to you has stopped breathing. The train is full of black smoke and you can see a fire.

THEME: ARTERIAL PULSES

Options

A Absent

B Alternans

C Bisferiens

D Collapsing

E Jerky

F Paradoxical

G Slow rising

For each of the conditions given below, choose the single arterial pulse characteristic that is likely to be encountered on physical examination from the list above. Each option may be used once, more than once or not at all.

☐ **1.12** **Aortic regurgitation.**

☐ **1.13** **Severe cardiac tamponade.**

☐ **1.14** **Severe left ventricular failure.**

☐ **1.15** **Aortic stenosis.**

☐ **1.16** **Takayasu arteritis.**

THEME: CLINICAL SIGNS OF STRUCTURAL HEART ABNORMALITIES

Options

A Atrial septal defect

B Aortic incompetence

C Aortic sclerosis

D Aortic stenosis

E Hypertrophic cardiomyopathy

F Left ventricular aneurysm

G Mitral incompetence

H Mitral stenosis

I Mitral valve prolapse

J Patent ductus arteriosus

K Pulmonary stenosis

L Tricuspid regurgitation

M Tricuspid stenosis

N Ventricular septal defect (VSD)

For each description of clinical signs below, choose the single most likely diagnosis from the list of options above. Each option may be used once, more than once or not at all.

☐ **1.17** There is a harsh pan-systolic murmur, loudest at the lower left sternal edge and inaudible at the apex. The apex is not displaced.

☐ **1.18** There is a soft late systolic murmur at the apex, radiating to the axilla.

☐ **1.19** The pulse is slow rising and the apex, which is not displaced, is heaving in character. There is an ejection systolic murmur heard best at the right second interspace that does not radiate.

☐ **1.20** The pulse is regular and jerky in character. The cardiac impulse is hyperdynamic and not displaced. There is a mid-systolic murmur, with no ejection click, loudest at the left sternal edge.

☐ **1.21** There is a constant 'machinery-like' murmur throughout systole and diastole.

THEME: MANAGEMENT OF HYPERLIPIDAEMIA

Options

A   Cholestyramine
B   Diet: fat intake < 30% of calories, with < 10% as saturated fat
C   Diet: fat intake < 25% of calories, with < 7% as saturated fat
D   Fibrate
E   Fibrate and statin
F   Nicotinic acid
G   No specific treatment required
H   Statin
I   Treat the secondary cause first

For each of the patients below, choose the first choice treatment from the list of options above. Each option may be used once, more than once or not at all. (Where a drug is recommended, you should assume that dietary advice is also given.)

☐ 1.22 A 60-year-old woman, recently diagnosed as having type 2 diabetes, is found to have a fasting total cholesterol level of 4.9 mmol/l and triglyceride level of 4.0 mmol/l. After 6 months of dietary treatment, her diabetes is well controlled but her triglyceride level is still 3.8 mmol/l.

☐ 1.23 A 70-year-old man has had an acute inferior myocardial infarction. On discharge, his total cholesterol level is 5.0 mmol/l and triglyceride level is 2.5 mmol/l.

☐ 1.24 A 40-year-old woman has symptomatic primary biliary cirrhosis. Her total cholesterol level is 7.8 mmol/l and triglyceride level is 2.1 mmol/l.

☐ 1.25 A 35-year-old man was admitted with acute pancreatitis. After he has recovered his triglyceride level is found to be 7.4 mmol/l. His cholesterol level is 6.7 mmol/l. He admits to drinking four cans of strong lager every day.

☐ **1.26** A 52-year-old man has peripheral vascular disease and angina. He has no secondary causes of dyslipidaemia. His total cholesterol level is 5.8 mmol/l and his triglyceride level is 3.4 mmol/l.

THEME: CARDIOLOGY IN CHILDREN

Options

A   Admit immediately to a paediatric unit

B   Chest X-ray

C   Electrocardiogram

D   Follow-up appointment

E   Ignore the findings

F   Routine outpatient appointment

For each of the patients below, choose the single most appropriate management option from the list of options above. Each option may be used once, more than once or not at all.

☐ **1.27** A 6-year-old visits her GP with fever and earache. On examination she looks well but is febrile and has otitis media. It is also noted that there is a quiet systolic murmur localised to the left sternal edge. Otherwise cardiac examination is normal.

☐ **1.28** A 6-week-old baby presents with difficulty feeding and poor weight gain. On examination the baby is tachypnoeic and tachycardic. There is a loud systolic murmur, intercostal recession and hepatomegaly.

☐ **1.29** A 3-day-old baby presents to accident and emergency with central cyanosis. There is a systolic murmur but otherwise the cardiovascular examination is normal.

☐ **1.30** During a routine 8-week baby check, the GP hears a loud pansystolic murmur at the left sternal edge. Otherwise the examination is normal and the baby is asymptomatic and thriving.

1.31   A 75-year-old man is found to have an irregular heartbeat. His electrocardiogram (ECG) shows repeating sequences of increasing PR interval followed by a dropped ventricular complex.

Choose the single most likely diagnosis from the options below.

- [ ] **A**   First-degree heart block
- [ ] **B**   Mobitz type I second-degree heart block
- [ ] **C**   Mobitz type II second-degree heart block
- [ ] **D**   Third-degree heart block
- [ ] **E**   Sick sinus syndrome

1.32   A 72-year-old man has heart failure and chronic obstructive pulmonary disease (COPD). He has come for his medication to be reviewed. His current medications are aspirin, lisinopril, simvastatin and inhalers for his COPD.

Which one other medication would he most benefit from?

- [ ] **A**   Amlodipine
- [ ] **B**   Bisoprolol
- [ ] **C**   Digoxin
- [ ] **D**   Losartan
- [ ] **E**   Ramipril

1.33   A 63-year-old woman with hypertension and recently diagnosed thyrotoxicosis complains of recent-onset palpitations. She is worried that the new medication she is taking for her thyrotoxicosis is causing these symptoms.

Which one of the following is the single most likely diagnosis in this patient?

- [ ] **A**   Atrial fibrillation
- [ ] **B**   Heart block
- [ ] **C**   Heart failure
- [ ] **D**   Side-effect of carbimazole
- [ ] **E**   Ventricular ectopics

ANSWERS

THEME: CHEST PAIN

1.1   A   Coronary artery spasm

Cocaine causes agitation, tachycardia, hypertension, arrhythmias and coronary artery spasm. Coronary artery spasm may lead to angina-type chest pain and even myocardial infarction.

1.2   B   Dissection of thoracic aorta

Dissection of the aorta within the chest causes severe central pain, that usually radiates to the back between the scapulae. Dissection of the aorta is associated with hypertension and collagen disorders (Marfan syndrome, pseudoxanthoma elasticum). Late-stage syphilis is also associated with dissection.

1.3   J   Pulmonary embolism

Antiphospholipid syndrome predisposes to recurrent thromboses. In this woman, a clot from her leg has embolised to the lung and caused infarction. The clinical presentation of pulmonary embolism ranges from mild pleuritic chest pain to cardiac arrest. Patients are often mildly short of breath and hypoxic on arterial blood gas testing and D-dimer testing will be positive. Chest X-rays are often normal. Diagnosis is by ventilation/perfusion scanning or spiral computed tomography.

1.4   K   Tietze disease

This disorder is caused by inflammation around the costosternal junctions. It may be bilateral or unilateral and the chest wall is very tender over the affected area. Reassurance and non-steroidal anti-inflammatory drugs (NSAIDs) are the mainstays of treatment.

1.5   D   Mesothelioma

This patient has long-standing pleural plaques, a sign of major previous asbestos exposure. Asbestos has many adverse effects on the lung, including pleural thickening (plaques), pleural effusions, fibrosis and mesothelioma. It is also associated with carcinoma of the bronchus. No medical treatment is known to alter the progress of asbestos-related disease.

1.6   C   Gastro-oesophageal reflux disease

This woman has reflux of gastric contents into the oesophagus, the acid nature of which is irritating the oesophageal mucosa and causing pain. This is often an indigestion-type pain, which may be relieved by antacids or proton pump inhibitors. Obesity, fatty foods, alcohol, cigarette smoking and large meals are associated with symptomatic disease. Complications include oesophageal stricture and Barrett oesophagus.

THEME: BASIC LIFE SUPPORT MANAGEMENT

1.7   B   Check pulse

In a cardiac arrest in a child, the recommendation is first to open the airway, then to check breathing. If the child is not breathing, five effective rescue breaths are given. After this, a central pulse should be checked. If this is absent then external cardiac massage is started. Alternate between breaths and cardiac massage at a ratio of 15:2 for two trained personnel, or 30:2 for lone rescuers. Continue for 1 minute. After this obtain access to advanced life support. You may be able to carry the child to a telephone if no-one else has summoned help. In reality, in a supermarket help will be on its way. In this case you continue CPR until help arrives or you become exhausted. (www.resus.org.uk/pages/pbls.pdf)

1.8   E   Leave patient

The most likely cause of a respiratory arrest in this adult patient is a cardiac arrest. The best chance of a successful outcome is if the patient is in ventricular fibrillation and is electrically defibrillated. In this situation you should leave the patient to summon help beofre starting basic life support. (www.resus.org.uk/pages/bls.pdf).

1.9   G   Place in recovery position

Groaning implies return of spontaneous breathing, and also adequate circulation. However, the man has a reduced level of consciousness. If he is lying on his back there is a danger of the tongue blocking the airway so he should be placed in the recovery position.

1.10   E   Leave patient

Rescue from drowning is an indication to start CPR rather than leaving the patient to summon help and a defibrillator. If there has been no response to initial CPR, leave the patient to get help. In an adult who may have sustained trauma or whose condition indicates drowning as the cause of cardiac arrest, the first action is also to give 1 minute of CPR prior to leaving to summon help. (www.resus.org.uk/pages/bls.pdf).

1.11   E   Leave patient

Your own safety is at risk. There is no merit in becoming another victim.

THEME: ARTERIAL PULSES

1.12   D   Collapsing

The upstroke is abrupt and steep. The peak of the wave form is reached earlier than normal and the downstroke is rapid. With a collapsing pulse the pulse pressure is greater than diastolic pressure. A collapsing pulse may also be found in patients with patent ductus arteriosus or an arteriovenous fistula.

1.13   F   Paradoxical

A paradoxical pulse (ie weakens in inspiration) also occurs in left ventricular compression, constrictive pericarditis or severe asthma.

1.14   B   Alternans

Pulsus alternans or alternating pulses describes a pulse with a regular rhythm but with alternating weak and strong beats. It is found in patients with severe heart failure and suggests a poor prognosis, ie prolonged recovery of the failing heart muscles.

1.15   G   Slow rising

A pulse that is slow rising and plateaus is found in moderate or severe aortic stenosis.

1.16   A   Absent

This idiopathic arteritis typically affects women between the ages of 20 and 40 years. It results in the narrowing of major arteries such as the renal, carotid, innominate and subclavian as well as the adjacent aorta. Cardiovascular examination may reveal absent pulses, aortic regurgitation, systolic murmurs above and below the clavicle and hypertension if the renal arteries are involved. Other causes of an absent radial pulse include trauma, dissection of the aorta with subclavian involvement, peripheral arterial embolus and post-catheterisation iatrogenic damage.

THEME: CLINICAL SIGNS OF STRUCTURAL HEART ABNORMALITIES

1.17 N Ventricular septal defect

The amplitude of a murmur depends on the amount of turbulence or flow. A small VSD (maladie de Roger) is louder than a large one. With a small VSD the pressure in the left ventricle is higher than the right so there is high flow per cross-sectional area of the defect. In a large VSD, ventricular pressures may equalise and there will be no flow across the defect. Reversal of the direction of flow (ie a right-to-left shunt) may occur, precipitating cyanosis and breathlessness. This is Eisenmenger syndrome and may occur acutely or chronically.

1.18 I Mitral valve prolapse

Late systolic murmurs that otherwise resemble mitral incompetence are usually due to mitral valve prolapse but may also be due to mild mitral incompetence (usually secondary to prolapse in such cases). There may also (or only) be a mid-systolic click. Clinical identification is important, as most cardiologists advise endocarditis prophylaxis for patients with mitral valve prolapse if it is clinically apparent, but not if it is an echo-only diagnosis.

1.19 D Aortic stenosis

This is the classic description of aortic stenosis. As the gradient increases the murmur gets louder and the pulse pressure becomes lower. There may also be postural hypotension. As the left ventricle fails, however, the murmur becomes softer as the flow through the valve is reduced.

1.20 E Hypertrophic cardiomyopathy

This is a classic description of hypertrophic cardiomyopathy. The hypertrophic septum causes functional obstruction of the left ventricular outflow tract (subaortic stenosis) and produces a murmur similar to aortic stenosis except that the second heart sound is normal.

1.21   J   Patent ductus arteriosus

Patent ductus arteriosus is now almost always identified and treated in the neonatal period. The murmur, when heard, is usually characteristic.

THEME: MANAGEMENT OF HYPERLIPIDAEMIA

These questions and answers are based on the British Hyperlipidaemia Association (BHA) guidelines.[1] Primary hypercholesterolaemia without other modifiable cardiovascular risk factors should be managed with diet restriction in the first instance. The BHA recommends two levels of dietary fat restriction, reserving the step 2 diet (answer C) for patients who have not reached desired cholesterol levels with step 1 diet (answer B). All patients with total cholesterol > 5.2 mmol/l and/or a triglyceride level > 2.3 mmol/l should be advised to follow at least a step 1 diet.

1.22   D   Fibrate

Undiagnosed or under-treated diabetes leads to high lipid levels, particularly triglycerides. Good diet and blood sugar control will often reduce triglyceride levels to an acceptable level. If diet fails, the treatment of choice for isolated hypertriglyceridaemia is a fibrate. Nicotinic acid is an alternative if fibrates are not tolerated. In mixed hyperlipidaemia, the treatment of choice is a fibrate or atorvastatin.

1.23   H   Statin

There is good evidence that statins prescribed after myocardial infarction reduce cardiovascular mortality. This benefit seems to extend to patients with 'normal' cholesterol levels. A rough target is a level of 4.5 mmol/l or less for total cholesterol. It should also be borne in mind that total cholesterol levels are falsely lowered from about 24 hours to 6 weeks after a myocardial infarction. A statin is usually prescribed without first attempting a trial of diet.

[1] DJ Betteridge, PM Doolson, PN Dunnington et al. 'Management of hyperlipidaemia: guidelines of the British Hyperlipidaemia Association'. *Postgraduate Medical Journal.* 1993, 69 359–369.

1.24   A   Cholestyramine

Dyslipidaemia is common in patients with primary biliary cirrhosis, who often develop xanthomata and xanthelasma. There is no cure for primary biliary cirrhosis, so the lipids must be corrected actively. Cholestyramine binds bile salts and is used to treat pruritus associated with the disease. It is also reasonably effective in reducing cholesterol levels, but it may cause a rise in triglycerides. Dietary restriction should also be advised.

1.25   I   Treat the secondary cause first

Excess alcohol may cause dyslipidaemia even in the absence of cirrhosis. Triglycerides are more likely to be raised than cholesterol but both may occur. Cessation of drinking will often reduce both lipids to normal levels without specific treatment. However, compliance with abstinence is often poor.

1.26   B   Diet: fat intake < 30% of calories, with < 10% as saturated fat

This patient has established vascular disease and mixed dyslipidaemia at a moderate level. Dietary advice should be given in the first instance but there should be a low threshold for medical treatment, probably a statin. Many physicians would immediately start a statin. The Quality and Outcomes Framework (QOF) guidelines in general practice recommend giving a statin to all patients with known cardiovascular disease (secondary prevention).

THEME: CARDIOLOGY IN CHILDREN

1.27   D   Follow-up appointment

This is likely to be an innocent murmur, which up to a third of children have at some point. They are not associated with any structural abnormality. The features of an innocent murmur are a quiet systolic murmur at the left sternal edge with no radiation. There is no diastolic component and no thrill. The child is otherwise asymptomatic and thriving. These murmurs are common during a febrile illness, due to the increased cardiac output.

1.28   A   Admit immediately to a paediatric unit

This baby has signs and symptoms suggestive of heart failure. The other common symptoms are sweating and recurrent chest infections. This baby needs an urgent assessment by a paediatrician. An electrocardiogram (ECG) and chest X-ray may help with diagnosing the underlying cause.

1.29   A   Admit immediately to a paediatric unit

This baby may have a duct-dependent cardiac defect. When the ductus arteriosus closes in the first few days of life the baby will become symptomatic, and survival will then balance on maintaining the patency of the duct with prostaglandin. This is a paediatric emergency and the baby needs to be assessed urgently by a paediatrician.

1.30   F   Routine outpatient appointment

This baby may have a ventricular septal defect. This is the commonest congenital heart defect. It is often picked up incidentally at a routine examination. The defect often closes spontaneously in the first week of life. As the baby is well they can be seen in an outpatient clinic. For the meantime, you should tell the parents about the signs of heart failure and to seek help if they occur.

1.31   B   Mobitz type I second-degree heart block

This abnormal pattern of conduction through the atrioventricular node (AV) node is also known as 'Wenckebach' type. The AV node becomes increasingly refractory to conduction, with an increasing PR interval on the ECG, until there is complete failure of conduction across the AV node and a QRS complex is dropped. Ischaemic heart disease and fibrosis of the conduction fibres in elderly people are the commonest causes. In Mobitz type II block the PR interval is constant with a regular dropped beat.

1.32   B   Bisoprolol

COPD is not an absolute contraindication to β-blocker treatment. In cases where up-titration is difficult, results from studies indicated that in terms of mortality and symptoms, some β-blocker is better than no β-blocker. Sometimes initiation of β-blockers is done in secondary care so the patient may need to be referred back to the hospital for this. Temporary exacerbation of symptoms may occur in 20–30% of patients when treatment with β-blockers is started, which may require increasing the dose of diuretic treatment.

1.33   A   Atrial fibrillation

Atrial fibrillation is the most likely cause of this patient's palpitations. Thyrotoxicosis can precipitate atrial fibrillation. It is important that she is given medication to control the heart rate, and anticoagulation should be considered. As the thyrotoxicosis improves, the atrial fibrillation may well improve or the patient may even revert back to sinus rhythm.

Chapter 2
Dermatology,
ENT and Eye

QUESTIONS

THEME: ACUTE RED EYE

Options

A Acute glaucoma

B Central retinal vein occlusion

C Conjunctivitis

D Dacryocystitis

E Episcleritis

F Iritis

G Keratitis

H Scleritis

I Subconjunctival haemorrhage

For each of the clinical scenarios below, choose the single most likely diagnosis from the list of options above. Each option may be used once, more than once or not at all.

☐ **2.1** Bilateral itchy red eyes with profuse watery discharge but with normal visual acuity. The tarsal conjunctiva reveals a follicular appearance.

☐ **2.2** Painful red eye with a mucopurulent discharge. There is circumcorneal redness, with a hypopyon and a white opacity of the cornea.

☐ **2.3** Unilateral red eye with pain, photophobia and mild reduction in visual acuity, and a small pupil.

☐ **2.4** Severely painful red eye in an elderly man with reduced visual acuity, nausea and vomiting. The pupil is fixed and semi-dilated. There is intense engorgement of the corneal and episcleral vessels with corneal oedema.

☐ **2.5** Acute painful erythema limited to the inferolateral quadrant of the eye in a 35-year-old woman.

THEME: DIAGNOSIS OF RASHES

Options

A Behçet's syndrome

B Contact dermatitis

C Dermatitis herpetiformis

D Eczema

E Lichen planus

F Pityriasis rosea

G Pityriasis versicolor

H Psoriasis

I Scabies

J Vitiligo

For each of the clinical scenarios given below, choose the single most likely diagnosis from the list of options above. Each option may be used once, more than once or not at all.

☐ **2.6** Intense pruritus worse at night and a non-specific excoriated rash for 1 month. The patient's partner also has itching.

☐ **2.7** Pink oval macules on the trunk with peripheral scaling, preceded by a larger patch the week before.

☐ **2.8** Depigmented patches on the trunk with fine scale that have appeared in a white patient after a holiday in the sun.

☐ **2.9** Red scaly plaques on the knees.

☐ **2.10** Itchy small blisters on the shoulders with raw areas caused by scratching. The patient has coeliac disease.

THEME: FACIAL RASHES

Options

A   Acne rosacea

B   Addison disease

C   Chloasma

D   Discoid lupus erythematosus

E   Lupus pernio

F   Lupus vulgaris

G   Mitral stenosis

H   Peutz–Jeghers syndrome

I   Rhinophyma

J   Seborrhoeic dermatitis

K   Systemic lupus erythematosus

For each of the following scenarios, choose the single most likely cause for the facial rash from the list of options above. Each option may be used once, more than once or not at all.

☐ **2.11**   A 25-year-old man has excessive dandruff and a pruritic erythematous rash affecting his eyebrows, ears, scalp and lateral margins of the nose.

☐ **2.12**   A 35-year-old woman with a malar butterfly rash complains of a dry mouth and joint pains.

☐ **2.13**   A 40-year-old woman has a diffuse, purple-red infiltration of the nose and cheeks. She has had a persistent dry cough, mild dyspnoea, weight loss and malaise for over a year. Chest examination appears normal.

☐ **2.14**   A patient presents to the accident and emergency department with recurrent colicky abdominal pain. There are several small brownish-black macules on the perioral skin and oral mucosa.

☐ **2.15**   A 45-year-old man presents with a persistent reddish papulopustular rash affecting the cheeks, nose, forehead and chin. The nose appears bulbous and craggy.

THEME: HAIR LOSS

Options

A Alopecia areata

B Androgenetic alopecia

C Colchicine

D Hypothyroidism

E Iron deficiency

F Lichen planus

G Lupus erythematosus

H Malnutrition

I Psoriasis

J Scalp ringworm

K Secondary syphilis

L Telogen effluvium

M Traumatic

For each of the following scenarios, choose the single most likely diagnosis from the list of options above. Each option may be used once, more than once or not at all.

☐ **2.16** A 55-year-old woman is complaining of patchy hair loss with localised areas of erythema, scaling and scarring affecting the scalp. She has a sore mouth and a skin rash affecting the flexor surfaces of her wrists and shins.

☐ **2.17** A 20-year-old man presents with sharply defined non-erythematous patches of baldness on his scalp. His eyebrows and beard are also affected. In the affected areas there are a few broken off stubby hairs that taper towards the scalp.

☐ **2.18** Three months after a severe illness with high temperature, an 18-year-old man notices excessive numbers of hairs in his hairbrush and on his pillow.

2.19   A 50-year-old woman notices some diffuse thinning of her hair with bitemporal recession.

2.20   A 10-year-old boy has a scaly patch on the scalp with numerous broken-off hairs.

THEME: SKIN DISEASE IN CHILDREN

Options

A Erythema chronicum migrans

B Erythema infectiosum

C Erythema multiforme

D Erythema nodosum

E Exanthema subitum

F Purpura fulminans

G Tinea corporis

For each of the clinical scenarios given below, choose the condition most associated with each from the list of options above. Each option may be used once, more than once or not at all.

☐ **2.21** A 9-month-old infant has been non-specifically unwell for 3 days with a fever. The rash subsides and the infant breaks out in a maculopapular rash over his body.

☐ **2.22** Following a course of penicillin for a bacterial infection, a 5-year-old child breaks out in a widespread macular rash with target lesions.

☐ **2.23** A 4-year-old boy has a runny nose and mild fever and develops bright red cheeks and reticular rash on the forearms.

☐ **2.24** Following a tick bite on holiday in a forested area, a 7-year-old boy develops an erythematous macule at the site of the bite, which then spreads to form an annular lesion with a clear central area.

THEME: INVESTIGATION OF LUMPS IN THE NECK

Options

A   Doppler ultrasound

B   Digital subtraction angiography

C   Excision biopsy

D   Fine needle aspiration

E   Iodine uptake scan

F   Nasopharyngoscopy

G   Paul Bunnell test

H   Sialogram

I   Technetium scan

J   Thyroid function tests

K   Ultrasound

For each of the patients below, choose the most discriminatory investigation from the list of options above. Each option may be used once, more than once or not at all.

☐ **2.25**   A 53-year-old woman presents with a 6-month history of a mass below the angle of the jaw on the right. It is gradually increasing in size and is mobile and firm to the touch. There is no associated pain or facial weakness.

☐ **2.26**   A 68-year-old man presents with a mass in the anterior triangle of the neck. It has increased in size over the past 2 months. It is soft, pulsatile and there is an associated bruit.

☐ **2.27**   A 38-year-old woman presents with a 2-month history of a swelling in the anterior part of the neck, towards the left of the midline. The swelling is not painful and she feels otherwise well. On examination, she has a solitary thyroid nodule in the left lobe of the thyroid. She is clinically euthyroid.

☐ **2.28** A 46-year-old woman presents with a diffuse swelling in the anterior part of the neck. She also complains of a hoarse voice. On examination, she has a diffuse multinodular goitre, bradycardia and slow-relaxing reflexes.

☐ **2.29** A 27-year-old man complains of an intermittent painful swelling below his jaw. The pain and swelling is worse on eating. He is otherwise well. On examination, there is a small, tender swelling in the left submandibular region.

☐ **2.30** A 72-year-old man presents with a hard, painless swelling in the anterior triangle of the neck. He has had a hoarse voice for 2 months. He is a lifelong smoker and drinks heavily.

2.31   A 55-year-old woman presents with some flaccid blisters in the front part of her chest. Some areas are red and weeping. A biopsy shows a superficial intraepidermal split just above the basal layer with acantholysis.

Which one of the following is the most likely diagnosis?

- ☐ **A**   Bullous pemphigoid
- ☐ **B**   Dermatitis herpetiformis
- ☐ **C**   Epidermolysis bullosa
- ☐ **D**   Pemphigus vulgaris
- ☐ **E**   Tuberous sclerosis

2.32   A 5-year-old girl presents at the accident and emergency department with a severe sore throat, drooling of saliva, high temperature and stridor.

Which one of the following is the most appropriate management option?

- ☐ **A**   Call the ENT surgeon/senior anaesthetist to secure her airway
- ☐ **B**   Lie the child down and examine her throat with a spatula
- ☐ **C**   Take a lateral neck X-ray
- ☐ **D**   Prescribe a course of antibiotics and discharge the child
- ☐ **E**   Try to intubate the child immediately

2.33 A 5-year-old girl was taken to see her GP as her mother had noticed that she had developed a slight squint in her left eye. On examination, the red reflex is absent.

Which one of the following statements best describes this child's condition?

☐ **A** It has a very high mortality rate

☐ **B** Most cases present after the age of 3 years

☐ **C** The gene associated with this condition is located on chromosome 16

☐ **D** The pattern of inheritance is recessive

☐ **E** There is a significant risk of secondary malignancy in the survivors

2.34 A 76-year-old man presents with a lesion on the cheek. The lesion is ulcerated and has rolled-over edges. It has slowly enlarged over a 12-month period.

Which one of the following is the most likely diagnosis?

☐ **A** Basal cell carcinoma

☐ **B** Keratoacanthoma

☐ **C** Melanoma

☐ **D** Solar keratosis

☐ **E** Squamous cell carcinoma

ANSWERS

THEME: ACUTE RED EYE

2.1   C   Conjunctivitis

In viral conjunctivitis there is a watery discharge with tarsal follicles.

2.2   G   Keratitis

The cornea is an avascular, transparent structure. A breach in the corneal epithelium is necessary for infection to become established. Bacterial infection is associated with a mucopurulent discharge. A hypopyon is seen when pus cells accumulate in the anterior chamber of the eye. The white opacity is the corneal ulcer. The most important viral keratitis is herpetic, with the formation of a dendritic ulcer, which can usually only be seen after fluorescein staining.

2.3   F   Iritis

This is acute iritis. The inflammation predominantly involves the iris and ciliary body. The pupil is smaller than the unaffected side. A hypopyon may be seen in severe cases in which keratic precipitates (aggregates of cells on the posterior surface of the cornea) will be visible on slit lamp examination.

2.4   A   Acute glaucoma

The main features of acute glaucoma are decreased vision associated with severe pain and constitutional upset. This condition is most commonly seen in older patients with long-sightedness. It is important to measure intraocular pressures and administer pupil-constricting eye drops eg pilocarpine to open up the angle, as well as drugs such as acetazolamide to reduce the production of aqueous humour.

2.5   E   Episcleritis

Episcleritis is unilateral and frequently recurrent. It is more common in women aged 30–40 years. The redness is confined to one quadrant of the eye. A tender nodule may be present at the centre of the inflamed area. It may be associated with connective tissue disorders.

THEME: DIAGNOSIS OF RASHES

2.6   I   Scabies

Scabies is caused by infestation with the mite *Sarcoptes scabiei*. Always suspect scabies if the patient's contacts also have itching. The rash may vary from no rash to erythroderma. Search for linear or wavy burrows produced by the mites. They are most commonly found in the interdigital webs of the hands, and on the wrists and genitals.

2.7   F   Pityriasis rosea

The initial lesion is called a herald patch. The condition is possibly of viral origin and usually remits spontaneously. The lesions are sometimes itchy and can be treated with topical steroids.

2.8   G   Pityriasis versicolor

This is a fungal infection of the trunk caused by *Malassezia furfur*. There is depigmentation of tanned skin, but increased pigmentation of untanned skin. A topical imidazole such as miconazole cream can be used. Selenium shampoo can be applied to the skin overnight, which may speed up the treatment.

2.9   H   Psoriasis

There are many presentations of psoriasis, the most common being classic plaque psoriasis. Apart from the skin, psoriasis can affect the scalp, the nails and the joints.

2.10   C   Dermatitis herpetiformis

Dermatitis herpetiformis will benefit from a gluten-free diet. Oral dapsone is also used.

THEME: FACIAL RASHES

2.11   J   Seborrhoeic dermatitis

Seborrhoeic dermatitis may be associated with overgrowth of *Pityrosporum ovale*, a commensal yeast, and can be severe in patients with human immunodeficiency virus (HIV) disease. The eruption often affects sebaceous areas of the skin. Scalp and facial involvement is a common presentation in young men.

2.12   K   Systemic lupus erythematosus

Skin signs are present in approximately three-quarters of patients with systemic lupus erythematosus (SLE). The signs include facial butterfly rash, photosensitivity, round or oval discoid lesions, diffuse alopecia and vasculitis. The skin signs occur in association with involvement of other organs, as well as immunological abnormalities such as circulating antinuclear autoantibodies. In discoid lupus erythematosus (DLE), involvement is confined to the skin, with scaly round or oval red plaques appearing on the face, scalp or hands. Multisystem involvement is not a feature although 5% may subsequently develop SLE. Women are significantly more frequently affected in SLE (female:male ratio of up to 9:1) but in DLE the ratio drops to 2:1.

2.13   E   Lupus pernio

Sarcoidosis may affect the skin in up to a third of cases. The skin changes are variable. On the face there may be violaceous or brownish red papules and the term lupus pernio may be used to describe dusky-red infiltrated plaques on the nose. There may be associated erythema nodosum, with bilateral hilar lymphadenopathy. Chest examination may be normal. Treatment involves intralesional steroids or if there is significant internal organ involvement oral steroids, or methotrexate may be used. Lupus vulgaris describes the cutaneous form of tuberculosis and occurs in people with a moderate to high degree of immunity. The soft reddish-brown plaques commonly occur on facial or neck skin and tend to be associated with scarring.

2.14   H   Peutz–Jeghers syndrome

Peutz-Jeghers syndrome is a rare autosomal dominant condition in which affected patients have lentigines around and in the mouth and on the fingers as well as small and large bowel polyps. The bowel polyps can cause intestinal obstruction and rarely undergo malignant change.

2.15   A   Acne rosacea

Rosacea is a chronic inflammatory facial skin disorder of unknown aetiology. It is characteristically erythematous and pustular. It is commonest in middle age and in men may be associated with rhinophyma, that is to say hyperplasia of the connective tissue and sebaceous glands of the nose. Topical metronidazole gel and tetracyclines may be helpful.

THEME: HAIR LOSS

2.16   F   Lichen planus

Both lichen planus and lupus erythematosus can lead to scarring alopecia in addition to other cutaneous involvement. The lesions may respond to topical or intralesional corticosteroids or systemic treatment.

2.17   A   Alopecia areata

Alopecia areata is a common autoimmune condition that may start in the second or third decade. It presents with sharply defined areas of alopecia that are non-erythematous. The eyebrows and beard may also be involved. The nails may show pitting. Classically so-called exclamation-mark hairs are found in affected areas and taper towards the scalp.

2.18   L   Telogen effluvium

Childbirth, high temperature, illness and other stresses may result in synchronisation of the growth cycles of all the scalp hair follicles into the telogen resting mode, with uniform shedding of hair 3 months later.

2.19   B   Androgenetic alopecia

The so-called male pattern of hair loss or androgenetic hair loss may also occur in women, particularly after the menopause. They may have the typical male pattern of hair loss with bitemporal recession and a bald crown, or diffuse thinning of the hair. Minoxidil may stimulate some regrowth in a third of patients. Androgen-secreting tumours in women may present with virilisation and male pattern baldness.

2.20   J   Scalp ringworm

Hair loss with scaly scalp particularly should always raise the possibility of scalp ringworm (*Tinea capitis*). A variety of dermatophyte fungi can cause the infection, the amount of inflammation depending on the type. The diagnosis is confirmed by examination of skin scrapings. Treatment is by systemic antifungal agents such as griseofulvin and terbinafine, although the latter is not licensed for use in children. Treatment should be initiated early as hair loss may be permanent. Psoriasis of the scalp does not usually lead to alopecia.

CHAPTER 2 ANSWERS

THEME: SKIN DISEASE IN CHILDREN

2.21   E   Exanthema subitum

The pattern of rash is characteristic of roseola infantum and the rash is exanthema subitum. The causative agent is most commonly human herpes virus 6.

2.22   C   Erythema multiforme

Erythema multiforme has a multitude of precipitating factors including bacterial infection (eg mycoplasma), viral infections (eg herpes simplex) and drugs, most commonly sulphonamides, but penicillin can also cause the rash. The target lesion is characteristic of the condition.

2.23   B   Erythema infectiosum

This is the slapped cheek syndrome or erythema infectiosum. It is due to parvovirus B19 infection and is usually a benign condition. In certain cases, especially in individuals with underlying haematological abnormalities, it can result in aplastic crises.

2.24   A   Erythema chronicum migrans

A tick bite from areas inhabited by deer can resulted in *Borrelia* infection (Lyme disease). The disease progresses in stages. Initially there is the characteristic rash of erythema chronicum migrans. Complications include meningoencephalitis, muscloskeletal pain and cardiac abnormalities.

THEME: INVESTIGATION OF LUMPS IN THE NECK

2.25   C   Excision biopsy

Unilateral parotid swelling is usually due to a pleomorphic adenoma (mixed parotid tumour). It may be indistinguishable from carcinoma clinically, although carcinoma is usually painful, rapidly growing and may cause facial nerve palsy. Excision biopsy provides diagnosis and treatment. An incomplete biopsy may seed the tumour in the wound.

2.26   B   Digital subtraction angiography

A pulsatile mass in the neck is either due to a carotid artery aneurysm or a carotid body tumour (chemodectoma). The latter is usually firm but may be soft and pulsatile. Diagnosis may be made with Doppler ultrasound or digital subtraction angiography, which is the more discriminatory test. Do not go anywhere near these masses with a needle!

2.27   D   Fine needle aspiration

A solitary thyroid nodule may be benign or malignant; secretory or non-secretory; solid or cystic; and may be 'hot' or 'cold' (depending on uptake of radio-labelled iodine). Many cold nodules are malignant but may be non-secretory adenomas. Hot nodules are usually adenomas but rarely could be follicular carcinomas. On ultrasound, cystic nodules are usually benign, solid ones may be malignant. No single radiological investigation is diagnostic. Tissue diagnosis is required for any nodule unless it is hot and cystic, or the patient is thyrotoxic. Therefore the most discriminatory test is fine needle aspiration cytology. Proceeding straight to excision biopsy will mean that many benign lesions are removed unnecessarily and that some malignant lesions are not excised completely.

CHAPTER 2 ANSWERS

2.28   K   Ultrasound

Multinodular goitre may occur in association with hyperthyroidism or, rarely, hypothyroidism. It is most commonly associated with a euthyroid state. Ultrasound will confirm the typical multinodular architecture to establish the diagnosis. Multiple nodules do not require histological investigation, as they are almost never malignant. Thyroid function tests will help guide treatment.

2.29   H   Sialogram

Salivary gland stones most commonly occur in the submandibular gland. The clinical picture as given is classic in this condition. The stone may be palpable if it is in the duct. Confirmation of the diagnosis is made with plain X-ray or contrast sialography. Stones in the duct may be expressed bimanually; stones in the gland may require surgical excision.

2.30   F   Nasopharyngoscopy

Cervical lymphadenopathy may be the first and only clinical sign of an underlying carcinoma of the pharynx, larynx, head or neck. Any lymph node that cannot be otherwise explained must be investigated with this in mind. Direct nasopharyngoscopy should be performed as a bare minimum to identify any mucosal lesions. Occasionally the diagnosis may only be made after node biopsy reveals metastatic squamous cell carcinoma but the underlying cause is usually visible when it is looked for.

2.31   D   Pemphigus vulgaris

This occurs in the middle-aged population and affects both sexes equally. The blisters tend to rupture easily because the intradermal split (due to autoantibody depositions) is high up in the epidermis. In bullous pemphigoid the split is at the level of the basement membrane and the blisters remain for a longer period. Rarely, the disease can be drug induced (eg due to penicillamine or angiotensin-converting enzyme (ACE) inhibitors). Treatment is with very-high-dose oral prednisolone.

2.32   A   Call the ENT surgeon/senior anaesthetist to secure her airway

This is a clinical picture of acute epiglottitis. Trying to examine the child or trying to intubate, if you are not very experienced, may precipitate airway obstruction. The most appropriate management would be to ask for help from an experienced ENT surgeon/senior anaesthetist.

2.33   E   There is a significant risk of secondary malignancy in the survivors

Retinoblastoma accounts for about 5% of cases of severe visual impairment in children. The suspected gene is located on chromosome 13 and the mode of inheritance is dominant. Children from families that have the hereditary form should undergo regular screening. The commonest presentation is with a white papillary reflex or a squint. Treatment is with chemotherapy to shrink the tumour, followed by laser therapy to the retina to preserve vision. Although most patients are cured, many have impaired vision. There is a significant risk of secondary malignancy in survivors, especially sarcoma.

2.34   A   Basal cell carcinoma

Basal cell carcinomas are seen in the cheek area commonly above the line joining the angle of the mouth and the tragus. They are slow growing and rarely metastasise. The ulcerated basel cell ulcer (rodent ulcer) characteristically has a rolled border which is firm, smooth and pearly in appearance with telangiectasia.

Chapter 3
Endocrinology and Metabolic

QUESTIONS

THEME: BIOCHEMISTRY OF JAUNDICE

Options

A   Dubin–Johnson syndrome
B   Extrahepatic cholestasis
C   Gilbert syndrome
D   Haemolytic jaundice
E   Intrahepatic cholestasis
F   Long-term tricyclic antidepressant use

For each of the following set of laboratory results, choose the single most likely diagnosis from the list of options above. Each option may be used once, more than once or not at all.

☐ **3.1**   Mildly elevated serum bilirubin, normal haemoglobin, normal alkaline phosphatase, normal serum aspartate transaminase (AST). No urinary bilirubin.

☐ **3.2**   Elevated serum bilirubin with a very elevated alkaline phosphatase, minimally elevated AST, bilirubin in the urine, normal haemoglobin.

☐ **3.3**   Elevated serum bilirubin with a mildly elevated alkaline phosphatase and a very elevated AST, bilirubin in the urine, normal haemoglobin.

☐ **3.4**   Mildly elevated serum bilirubin, anaemia, normal alkaline phosphatase and AST. No urinary bilirubin.

THEME: UREA AND ELECTROLYTES

Options

A	Na⁺ 145	K⁺ 2.8	Ur 4.0	Cr 88
	Ca²⁺ 2.3	CK 39	Glu 4.7	
B	Na⁺ 141	K⁺ 3.9	Ur 6.2	Cr 60
	Ca²⁺ 2.29	CK 111	Glu 4.9	
C	Na⁺ 135	K⁺ 6.2	Ur 6.1	Cr 71
	Ca²⁺ 2.28	CK 122	Glu 5.1	
D	Na⁺ 142	K⁺ 6.4	Ur 16	Cr 158
	Ca²⁺ 2.3	CK 2210	Glu 4.5	
E	Na⁺ 154	K⁺ 5.9	Ur 21	Cr 160
	Ca²⁺ 2.25	CK 144	Glu 45	
F	Na⁺ 144	K⁺ 4.0	Ur 24	Cr 110
	Ca²⁺ 2.04	CK 123	Glu 9.6	

CHAPTER 3 QUESTIONS

Normal values

- Sodium (Na⁺) 135–145 mmol/l
- Potassium (K⁺) 3.5–5 mmol/l
- Urea (Ur) 2.5–6.7 mmol/l
- Creatinine (Cr) 70– < 150 mmol/l
- Calcium total (Ca²⁺) 2.12–2.65 mmol/l
- Creatinine kinase (CK): men 25–195 IU/l; women 25–170 IU/l
- Glucose fasting 3.5–6.0 mmol/l

From the options above, select the single most appropriate set of blood results that correspond with the cases described below. Each option may be used once, more than once or not at all.

☐ **3.5** A 78-year-old woman who is taking an angiotensin-converting enzyme (ACE) inhibitor and spironolactone to treat her worsening congestive cardiac failure is brought in with palpitations and a low blood pressure.

☐ **3.6** An elderly man is brought to the accident and emergency department by ambulance, having been found on the kitchen floor by his neighbour. He has been there all night, unable to get up.

☐ **3.7** A 23-year-old man has severe diarrhoea, having just returned from holiday. He is able to tolerate oral fluids.

☐ **3.8** A 23-year-old soldier who has been on a tough military exercise presents to the accident and emergency department with discoloured urine.

☐ **3.9** A 51-year-old man presents with severe epigastric pain going through to his back. It is constant in nature and he had a similar episode a year ago. He is known to be a heavy drinker. His electrocardiogram (ECG) is normal.

☐ **3.10** A semiconscious 66-year-old obese man is brought into the accident and emergency department. His cleaner found him unwell in bed. He takes bendroflumethiazide for his hypertension. It is known that he had diarrhoea and vomiting 2 days ago.

CHAPTER 3 QUESTIONS

THEME: ENDOCRINE DISEASE

Options

A Addison disease

B Conn syndrome

C Cushing syndrome

D Diabetes insipidus

E Graves disease

F Multiple endocrine neoplasia

G Phaeochromocytoma

H Syndrome of inappropriate antidiuretic hormone secretion

For each of the following clinical scenarios, choose the single most likely diagnosis from the list of options above. Each option may be used once, more than once or not at all.

☐ **3.11** A 56-year-old woman presents to the accident and emergency department with syncope. You notice she has a significant postural drop in blood pressure and also pigmentation in a recent scar on her neck.

☐ **3.12** A 48-year-old woman has developed striae on her abdomen and is hypertensive.

☐ **3.13** A 31-year-old woman has severe hypertension and is found to have a potassium level of 3.1 mmol/l.

☐ **3.14** A 32-year-old woman has a history of episodes of severe headache and anxiety with flushing. On examination she is very hypertensive and has a tachycardia.

THEME: ABNORMALITIES OF WATER AND ELECTROLYTE BALANCE

Options

A Addison disease

B Conn syndrome

C Diabetes insipidus

D Renal tubular acidosis

E *Salmonella enteritis*

F Thyrotoxicosis

For each set of blood chemistry results below, choose the single most likely diagnosis from the list of options above. Each option may be used once, more than once or not at all.

☐ **3.15**	Na 136 mmol/l	K 2.8 mmol/l	HCO_3 18 mmol/l
☐ **3.16**	Na 149 mmol/l	K 2.6 mmol/l	HCO_3 30 mmol/l
☐ **3.17**	Na 128 mmol/l	K 5.6 mmol/l	HCO_3 24 mmol/l
☐ **3.18**	Na 130 mmol/l	K 2.5 mmol/l	HCO_3 8 mmol/l
☐ **3.19**	Na 160 mmol/l	K 5.6 mmol/l	HCO_3 18 mmol/l

Normal values

- Sodium (Na): 135–145 mmol/l

- Potassium (K): 3.5–5 mmol/l

- Bicarbonate (HCO_3): 24–30 mmol/l

THEME: MANAGEMENT OF DIABETES MELLITUS

Options

A Acarbose

B Dietary modification

C Glibenclamide

D Gliclazide

E Intravenous insulin sliding scale

F Metformin

G No change in treatment required

H Once-daily long-acting insulin injection

I One long-acting and three short-acting insulin injections

J Repaglinide

K Subcutaneous insulin sliding scale

L Twice-daily long/short mixed insulin injections

For each of the patients below, choose the most appropriate next management step from the list of options above. Each option may be used once, more than once or not at all.

☐ **3.20** A 78-year-old woman is diagnosed as having diabetes after she was found to have a raised blood glucose level during an admission to hospital after a fall. Despite following appropriate dietary advice, her HbA1c remains elevated at 11%. She is not obese.

☐ **3.21** A 27-year-old woman was found to have glycosuria at a routine antenatal clinic visit. A glucose tolerance test confirms the diagnosis of gestational diabetes.

☐ **3.22** A 65-year-old man has had type 2 diabetes for 4 years, for which he is taking chlorpropamide. He is in hospital with an acute myocardial infarction and his laboratory blood glucose is 11 mmol/l.

☐ **3.23** A 58-year-old man was diagnosed as having diabetes at a routine medical examination 3 months ago. His body mass index is 32 kg/m^2 despite losing 5 kg by following the dietician's advice. His home blood glucose readings range from 7 mmol/l to 11 mmol/l and his HbA1c is 10%.

☐ **3.24** A 32-year-old woman has had type 1 diabetes for 15 years. She injects isophane insulin twice a day and rarely tests her blood glucose at home. You see her for the first time in over a year and find that she is 12 weeks' pregnant.

☐ **3.25** A 65-year-old man has had type 2 diabetes for 5 years. He is on the maximum dose of tolbutamide and metformin. All his home blood glucose readings are greater than 11 mmol/l and he complains of thirst and weight loss. His body mass index is 22 kg/m^2.

THEME: CALCIUM AND BONE

Options

A Acromegaly

B Hyperparathyroidism

C Multiple myeloma

D Osteomalacia

E Osteoporosis

F Paget disease

G Sarcoidosis

For each of the following clinical scenarios, choose the single most likely diagnosis from the list of options above. Each option may be used once, more than once or not at all.

☐ **3.26** A 45-year-old woman presents with nausea and vomiting. She also has been experiencing some left loin pain, which is worsening.

☐ **3.27** A 51-year-old man presents with nausea, vomiting and back pain. He has recently lost some weight. He is usually very fit and active.

☐ **3.28** A 78-year-old woman presents with sudden-onset severe back pain. She is otherwise well and has no other symptoms.

☐ **3.29** A 56-year-old African Caribbean patient present with nausea and vomiting associated with increased shortness of breath. He is usually very fit and well and is not taking any medications. He is also complaining of sore eyes.

3.30 A 26-year-old obese man presents to clinic. He is found to have a body mass index of 36 kg/m^2, and he wants advice about treatment of his obesity.

Which one of the following options pertains to the treatment of obesity?

- A Fenfluramine has now been banned in the UK because it causes systemic hypertension
- B Orlistat causes weight loss by inhibiting pancreatic and gastric lipase
- C The removal of large amounts of fat by liposuction tends to be quite effective in cases of sudden weight gain
- D Weight loss will be very slow at first when only glycogen breaks down, but this is followed 3–4 weeks later by a period of incremental weight loss due to the breakdown of adipose tissue
- E With morbid obesity in the under 18-year-old age group, restrictive surgery, which limits the size of the stomach so the person feels full after eating a small amount of food, may sometimes be tried before pharmacotherapy

3.31 A 23-year-old diabetic woman who depends on insulin comes to your clinic for pre-pregnancy counselling with regard to her glycaemic control and the right time to try for a baby.

Which one of the following options is the best test that will help you advise the patient?

- A 1-hour glucose tolerance test (GTT)
- B 2-hour GTT
- C HbA1c
- D Random blood sugar
- E Sugar series

3.32 A 36-year old woman regularly consumes about 40 units of alcohol.

Which one of the following statements about alcohol consumption is true?

☐ **A** 20% of people who regularly abuse alcohol develop liver cirrhosis

☐ **B** Alcohol dehydrogenase is most prevalent in the small intestine

☐ **C** 'Hangover' after drinking is a neurotoxic effect of alcohol

☐ **D** Occasional binges are more harmful than regular heavy drinking

☐ **E** Pregnant women should abstain only in the first trimester

3.33 Which one of the following is not associated with an increased risk of developing type 2 diabetes?

☐ **A** Age greater than 45 years

☐ **B** Central obesity

☐ **C** Family history of diabetes

☐ **D** History of gestational diabetes

☐ **E** Smoking

ANSWERS

THEME: BIOCHEMISTRY OF JAUNDICE

3.1   C   Gilbert syndrome

In Gilbert syndrome the bilirubin is unconjugated due to congenital failure of the hepatocytes to take up the bilirubin for conjugation. Therefore there is no bilirubin in the urine as only the conjugated form is water soluble and appears in the urine. Dubin–Johnson syndrome is the congenital failure of excretion of the conjugated bilirubin into the bile canaliculi.

3.2   B   Extrahepatic cholestasis

The very elevated alkaline phosphatase in the presence of jaundice indicates extrahepatic obstruction, typically from a common bile duct stone or carcinoma of the head of the pancreas.

3.3   E   Intrahepatic cholestasis

In intrahepatic cholestasis, the AST is very elevated but the alkaline phosphatase, which arises from the bile duct walls, is not. Common causes are drugs, alcohol and infective hepatitis.

3.4   D   Haemolytic jaundice

In haemolytic jaundice there will be anaemia. There is no elevation in urinary bilirubin because the haemolysis releases unconjugated bilirubin, which is not water soluble and therefore will not appear in the urine.

THEME: UREA AND ELECTROLYTES

3.5

C				
	Na$^+$ 135	K$^+$ 6.2	Ur 6.1	Cr 71
	Ca^{2+} 2.28	CK 122	Glu 5.1	

This woman is having runs of ventricular tachycardia and has associated low blood pressure. Both ACE inhibitors and spironolactone promote sodium excretion and potassium retention. This may lead to hyperkalaemia, which predisposes to ventricular arrhythmias. Her treatment should include calcium ions to stabilise the myocardium, and an insulin and dextrose infusion to promote the cellular uptake of intravascular potassium.

3.6

D				
	Na$^+$ 142	K$^+$ 6.4	Ur 16	Cr 158
	Ca^{2+} 2.3	CK 2210	Glu 4.5	

This elderly man has rhabdomyolysis secondary to pressure necrosis of his muscles, caused by the prolonged period of lying on the hard floor. His CK is high, due to its release from damaged muscle cells. Management must include adequate hydration to prevent renal failure, and treatment of hyperkalaemia. A cause for the initial fall must also be sought.

3.7

A				
	Na$^+$ 145	K$^+$ 2.8	Ur 4.0	Cr 88
	Ca^{2+} 2.3	CK 39	Glu 4.7	

This patient has hypokalaemia as a result of diarrhoea. He has been able to maintain hydration. Severe hypokalaemia causes muscle weakness, a decreased-amplitude electrocardiogram (ECG), a prolonged QT interval and, in extreme circumstances, it may lead to asystolic cardiac arrest.

3.8

D	Na⁺ 142	K⁺ 6.4	Ur 16	Cr 158
	Ca²⁺ 2.3	CK 2210	Glu 4.5	

This fit young soldier has developed rhabdomyolysis secondary to severe muscular exercise. Other causes include trauma, including prolonged pressure, and statin therapy for hypercholesterolaemia.

3.9

F	Na⁺ 144	K⁺ 4.0	Ur 24	Cr 110
	Ca²⁺ 2.04	CK 123	Glu 9.0	

This patient has acute pancreatitis. Serum amylase is usually greatly elevated in this condition. Patients are in severe pain, requiring opioid analgesia, and in cardiovascular shock resulting in raised level of urea. They have a raised white cell count, and may have increased blood glucose levels reflecting reduced pancreatic function. They also have an acute fall in serum albumin with a consequent fall in serum calcium.

3.10

E	Na⁺ 154	K⁺ 5.9	Ur 21	Cr 160
	Ca²⁺ 2.25	CK 144	Glu 45	

This patient has hyperosmolar non-ketotic coma (HONK). It is a condition that signifies a type 2 diabetic (non-insulin-dependent diabetes mellitus, NIDDM) emergency. Severe hyperglycaemia leads to profound dehydration and patients develop a hyperosmolar state (osmolality = $2([Na^+] + [K^+]) + [Glu] + [Urea]$). However, there is no ketosis in contrast to the diabetic emergency of ketoacidosis seen in type 1 diabetes. Due to the hyperosmolar state, patients often have a decreased level of consciousness on presentation.

THEME: ENDOCRINE DISEASE

3.11   A   Addison disease

Primary hypoadrenalism due to destruction of the adrenal cortex leads to a reduction in glucocorticoid, mineralocorticoid and sex steroid production. Reduced cortisol levels produce an increase in adrenocorticotropic hormone (ACTH) production by the pituitary, which is responsible for the pigmentation by its action on melanocytes. Postural hypotension is due to hypovolaemia and sodium loss.

3.12   C   Cushing syndrome

Cushing syndrome is due to an increase in the secretion of glucocorticoids. In Cushing disease there is an increase in ACTH production by the pituitary gland. Other causes are ACTH-producing tumours and non-ACTH dependent causes such as an adrenal adenoma.

3.13   B   Conn syndrome

Primary hyperaldosteronism causes sodium retention, hypertension and hypokalaemia. Conn syndrome is due to an adrenal adenoma, but adrenal hyperplasia can also cause the condition.

3.14   G   Phaeochromocytoma

Tumours that release noradrenaline and adrenaline (norepinephrine and epinephrine) frequently cause intermittent symptoms. Most phaeochromocytomas arise from the adrenal glands. Some are associated with the multiple endocrine neoplasia syndromes.

THEME: ABNORMALITIES OF WATER AND ELECTROLYTE BALANCE

3.15   D   Renal tubular acidosis

The hallmark of renal tubular acidosis is a mild metabolic acidosis with hypokalaemia. The normal range for serum bicarbonate concentration is 24–30 mmol/l. The low level suggests acidosis. The clinical picture is common after treatment with acetazolamide.

3.16   B   Conn syndrome

Conn syndrome or primary hyperaldosteronism is a rare condition, but it is important as a cause of secondary arterial hypertension. The main clinical feature is hypertension without oedema and the combination of mild hypernatraemia with hypokalaemia.

3.17   A   Addison disease

Addison disease or adrenal failure is characterised by low blood pressure, pigmentation of the skin and buccal mucosa, and the combination of hyponatraemia and mild hyperkalaemia.

3.18   E   *Salmonella enteritis*

Severe diarrhoea results in metabolic acidosis due to bicarbonate loss and hypokalaemia. (Remember: the bicarbonate content of bowel is approximately 80 mmol/l.)

3.19   C   Diabetes insipidus

Diabetes insipidus is due to antidiuretic hormone (ADH) deficiency or lack/loss of renal ADH responsiveness. These patients lose predominantly free water and present with polyuria and dehydration. Other causes of a similar electrolyte pattern are poor fluid intake or water loss due to fever/hyperventilation.

CHAPTER 3 ANSWERS

THEME: MANAGEMENT OF DIABETES MELLITUS

3.20   D   Gliclazide

This patient will almost certainly have type 2 diabetes. Diet alone will control the diabetes many of these patients. If that does not happen, the patient requires an oral hypoglycaemic agent. Biguanides (metformin) are the drug of choice if the patient is obese unless they have cardiac or renal failure. Sulphonylureas are the drugs of choice if the patient is not obese. In older patients, a short-acting agent minimises the risk of hypoglycaemia or drug accumulation if there is impairment of renal function. Glibenclamide and chlorpropamide are longest acting and, therefore, least safe. Gliclazide and tolbutamide are shorter acting and safer.

3.21   B   Dietary modification

Gestational diabetes (diabetes arising for the first time in pregnancy) is often treatable with diet control alone. The patient needs to be counselled well and must be encouraged to monitor blood glucose at home. A few women will require insulin to achieve glycaemic control. Oral hypoglycaemics should not be used in pregnancy. Glycosuria is common in pregnancy due to lowering of the renal threshold. If glycosuria is persistently present, a glucose tolerance test should be done. Some women with gestational diabetes either remain diabetic or subsequently develop diabetes.

3.22   E   Intravenous insulin sliding scale

There is good evidence that cardiac mortality is reduced with the use of insulin following myocardial infarction. Any patient with a known diagnosis of diabetes, regardless of treatment, or with a blood glucose greater than 8.0 mmol/l at presentation with an acute myocardial infarction should receive insulin treatment. The regimen used in the landmark trial was 3 days on an intravenous insulin sliding scale followed by 3 months on subcutaneous insulin. The subgroup of patients converted to insulin from sulphonylureas benefited the most.[2]

3.23   F   Metformin

This man's type 2 diabetes is inadequately controlled (preprandial blood glucose should be 4–7 mmol/l and HbA1c should be < 7.0%). Metformin is the drug of choice, as he is obese. If this fails, acarbose or a sulphonylurea may be tried.

3.24   I   One long-acting and three short-acting insulin injections

Pregnant women with diabetes have an increased risk of most maternal and fetal complications, and an increased risk of accelerated complication of diabetes. Particular risks are intrauterine death, premature labour, pre-eclampsia, congenital malformations and neonatal mortality. There is good evidence that tight glycaemic control improves outcome but at the expense of increasing the mother's risk of hypoglycaemia. A four times daily regimen (three injections of soluble insulin and one injection of long-acting insulin) has recently been shown to reduce the risk of hypoglycaemic attacks. The patient in this question will require considerable support and counselling.

3.25   H   Once-daily long-acting insulin injection

A patient with type 2 diabetes may require insulin if good glycaemic control cannot be achieved with diet and oral medication. If a patient is on metformin and a sulphonylurea and is obese, then acarbose or repaglinide may be tried. If they are not obese, insulin is required. Insulin may be given instead of oral medication. It is more usual to add a once-daily dose of long-acting insulin to the oral regimen. This patient is symptomatic so should probably receive insulin even if he were obese.

[2] K. Malmberg, L Ryden, A Hamsten et al. 'Randomized trial of insulin-glucose infusion followed by subcutaneous insultin treatment in diabetic patients with acute myocardial infarction (DIGAMI study): effects on mortality at 1 year'. Journal of the American College of Cardiology. 1995, 26: 56–65.

CHAPTER 3 ANSWERS

THEME: CALCIUM AND BONE

3.26   B   Hyperparathyroidism

Primary hyperparathyroidism is usually due to a single parathyroid adenoma. It may cause renal calculi. Treatment is by surgical excision of the underlying parathyroid tumour(s).

3.27   C   Multiple myeloma

This patient's symptoms of hypercalcaemia are due to excessive bone destruction. Bone pain, particularly back pain, is the commonest symptom of myeloma and is caused by vertebral collapse and nerve entrapment. Myeloma is diagnosed by the presence of a monoclonal protein, usually IgG or IgA, in the serum in 80% of cases. In the remainder, light chains (Bence Jones protein) can be detected in the urine.

3.28   E   Osteoporosis

A wedge fracture due to osteoporosis is the most likely diagnosis in this woman as she is otherwise asymptomatic. Many people with osteoporosis are unaware they have it until they present with a facture.

3.29   G   Sarcoidosis

Sarcoidosis is a systemic disease with non-caseating granuloma in lymph nodes and other sites. It is a recognised cause of hypercalcaemia and is more common in people of African Caribbean origin. It can be associated with anterior and posterior uveitis. Treatment is usually with corticosteroids.

3.30   B   Orlistat causes weight loss by inhibiting pancreatic and gastric lipase

According to the National Institute for Health and Clinical Excellence (NICE) guidance on obesity (www.nice.org.uk/guidance/CG43) people are considered to be morbidly obese if they have a body mass index of 40 kg/m² or more, or if they have a body mass index between 35 kg/m² and 40 kg/m² and other significant disease (for example, diabetes, high blood pressure) that may be improved if they lose weight. Weight loss occurs rapidly at the start and then slows down significantly. Surgery is contraindicated in children below the age of 18 years according to NICE guidelines. NICE recommends that surgery should be available as a treatment option provided that patients meet all of the following criteria:

- They are adults (aged 18 or over).

- They have a body mass index (BMI) of 40 kg/m² or more, or between 35 kg/m² and 40 kg/m² and other significant disease (for example, type 2 diabetes or high blood pressure) that could be improved if they lost weight.

- All appropriate non-surgical measures have been tried but the patient has not been able to achieve or maintain adequate, clinically beneficial weight loss for at least 6 months.

- The person has been receiving or will receive intensive management in a specialist obesity service.

- The person is generally fit for anaesthesia and surgery.

- The person is committed to long-term follow-up.

There are two main types of surgery to aid weight loss, known as 'malabsorptive' and 'restrictive' procedures. Malabsorptive surgery works by shortening the length of the digestive tract (gut) so that the amount of food absorbed by the body is reduced. In this type of surgery, a bypass is created by joining one part of the intestine to another. Restrictive surgery limits the size of the stomach so the person feels full after eating a small amount of food. This type of surgery can involve 'stapling' parts of the stomach together or fitting a tight band to make a small pouch for food to enter.

Orlistat inhibits pancreatic and gastric lipase, and works by inhibiting the absorption of fat from the diet. Patients need to cut down their intake of fat sufficiently to avoid diarrhoea.

Fenfluramine causes pulmonary hypertension and heart valve disease, which is why it has been banned.

3.31   C   HbA1c

This best measures the average blood glucose concentration over the lifespan of a haemoglobin molecule, which is approximately 6 weeks. Levels below 6% are considered to be a reflection of good glycaemic control and the patient can start trying for a baby at this stage. Folic acid supplementation is necessary because diabetic mothers have an increased risk of having babies with neural tube defects. And folic acid supplementation is a preventative measure.

3.32   A   20% of people who regularly drink alcohol develop liver cirrhosis

Autopsy reports indicate a high prevalence of cirrhosis in regular heavy drinkers, and the likelihood increases with the duration of the heavy drinking pattern. The clinical incidence of complications due to cirrhosis is somewhat lower. An intermittent 'binge drinking' pattern less commonly causes cirrhosis than the same overall alcohol consumption in regular drinking. However, binge drinking is associated with a higher incidence of cardiomyopathy, acute pancreatitis and accidental injury. Pregnant women should be advised to abstain from alcohol for the entire duration of pregnancy to minimise the risks of fetal alcohol syndrome and subsequent developmental delays in the newborn. Short-term adverse effects, including headache and nausea during 'hangover', are often caused by congeners such as isoamyl alcohol or metabolites such as acetaldehyde, rather than being a direct toxic effect of alcohol itself. Alcohol dehydrogenase is found in the stomach and liver.

3.33 E Smoking

All the other options are associated with an increased risk of developing type 2 diabetes. Patients with type 2 diabetes who smoke have a greatly increased risk of developing cardiovascular disease. The International Diabetes Federation has recently published a consensus statement which recommends that healthcare professionals should identify people at high risk of type 2 diabetes opportunistically.

Chapter 4
Gastroenterology and Nutrition

QUESTIONS

THEME: CAUSES OF CONSTIPATION

Options

A   Anal fissure

B   Bed rest

C   Bowel obstruction

D   Carcinoma of the colon

E   Carcinoma of the rectum

F   Depression

G   Hypercalcaemia

H   Hypothyroidism

I   Iatrogenic

J   Irritable bowel syndrome

K   Poor fibre intake

L   Pregnancy

For each of the patients below, choose the single most likely diagnosis from the list of options above. Each option may be used once, more than once or not at all.

☐ **4.1**   A 60-year-old woman presents with a 3-day history of constipation, colicky abdominal pain, distension and vomiting. She has not even passed wind. Bowel sounds are active and high pitched.

☐ **4.2**   A 30-year-old man complains of constipation and pain on defecation. He also notices small amounts of fresh blood on the paper afterwards. He is unable to tolerate a rectal examination.

☐ **4.3** A 21-year-old woman with mild learning difficulties complains of recent onset of abdominal distension, constipation, indigestion and amenorrhoea.

☐ **4.4** A 65-year-old man complains of constipation, low mood, low back pain that prevents him sleeping, fatigue and thirst. He has bony tenderness over his lumbar spine.

☐ **4.5** A 52-year-old woman complains of constipation and nausea 4 days after abdominal hysterectomy for fibroids. On examination she has active bowel sounds of normal pitch and pinpoint pupils.

☐ **4.6** A 60-year-old man presents with a 2-month history of increasing constipation with occasional diarrhoea. He also describes anorexia, weight loss and a feeling of tenesmus.

THEME: CAUSES OF HEPATOMEGALY

Options

A   Acute myeloid leukaemia

B   Amyloidosis

C   Congestive cardiac failure

D   Chronic lymphocytic leukaemia

E   Chronic myeloid leukaemia

F   Hepatocellular carcinoma

G   Infectious mononucleosis

H   Liver metastases

I   Lymphoma

J   Malaria

K   Myelofibrosis

L   Tricuspid regurgitation

For each of the patients below, choose the single most likely diagnosis from the list of options above. Each option may be used once, more than once or not at all.

☐ **4.7**   **A 20-year-old student presents to her GP with a 1-week history of fever and sore throat. On examination, she has tender cervical lymphadenopathy and an enlarged, tender liver.**

☐ **4.8**   **A 62-year-old man presents with a 3-month history of intermittent constipation and diarrhoea and progressive weight loss. On examination, he is cachectic and has knobbly hepatomegaly. He is not jaundiced. His liver function is normal.**

☐ **4.9** An 81-year-old woman presents with a 6-month history of abdominal swelling, hepatomegaly and leg oedema. She has a history of rheumatic fever as a child and hypertension for the past few years. She takes atenolol for her hypertension.

☐ **4.10** A 56-year-old woman has a 20-year history of rheumatoid arthritis. Despite numerous drugs, her arthritis has only recently been under control. Recently she has noticed that she bruises easily. On examination she has a large beefy tongue, lymphadenopathy and hepatomegaly.

☐ **4.11** A 31-year-old man presents to casualty with a 2-week history of night sweats, weight loss and pruritus. He has noticed some enlarged glands in his groin that become painful if he drinks alcohol. On examination he has no other evidence of lymphadenopathy but there is a smooth enlarged liver.

THEME: CAUSES OF DYSPHAGIA

Options

A Achalasia
B Bronchial carcinoma
C Carcinoma of the oesophagus
D Chronic benign stricture
E Left atrial hypertrophy
F Myasthenia gravis
G Oesophageal candidosis
H Pharyngeal pouch
I Plummer–Vinson syndrome
J Reflux oesophagitis
K Thoracic aneurysm

For each of the patients below, choose the most likely diagnosis from the list of options above. Each option may be used once, more than once or not at all.

☐ **4.12** A 50-year-old obese woman complains of a burning retrosternal discomfort after eating and on lying down. She has also noticed excessive salivation and wheezing when she lies down to sleep.

☐ **4.13** A 35-year-old housewife has noticed progressively worsening difficulty swallowing over several years. She has been troubled by regurgitation of undigested food and halitosis, and has fits of coughing on lying flat.

☐ **4.14** A 45-year-old pale woman complains that food is sticking in the back of her throat. On examination she has spoon-shaped nails, a smooth tongue and angular cheilitis.

☐ **4.15** A 65-year-old man complains of difficulty in swallowing. He finds that the first mouthful of food is easy to swallow but thereafter he has increasing difficulty in swallowing until he regurgitates undigested food. He also notices a neck swelling.

☐ **4.16** A 60-year-old woman complains of difficulty swallowing. On examination she has a prominent malar flush, an irregularly irregular pulse and raised jugular venous pressure. On auscultation there is a rumbling, long, low-pitched, mid-diastolic murmur best heard in the left lateral position in expiration.

THEME: ACUTE ABDOMEN

Options

A   Acute salpingitis

B   Adhesive small bowel obstruction

C   Appendicitis

D   Leaking aortic aneurysm

E   Mesenteric ischaemia

F   Pancreatitis

G   Perforated peptic ulcer

H   Torsion of an ovarian cyst

I   Ureteric colic

For each of the patients below, choose the single most likely diagnosis from the list of options above. Each option may be used once, more than once or not at all.

☐ **4.17**   A 60-year-old man with epigastric pain and brief collapse at home is now alert with some mild back pain and tachycardia.

☐ **4.18**   A 45-year-old man has been taking ibuprofen for persistent abdominal pain. He has been brought to accident and emergency after a sudden collapse, and an erect chest film shows gas under the diaphragm.

☐ **4.19**   A 36-year-old woman has been brought to accident and emergency by her husband with very severe left-sided abdominal pain. Her husband states that she has been pacing around the bedroom all night, unable to find a comfortable position, and the patient describes the pain as being 'worse than a labour pain'.

☐ **4.20** An 87-year-old woman is admitted with a rigid abdomen. A careful history reveals she has been having pain after meals and has stopped eating very much. Her blood gas assay reveals a metabolic acidosis. Her amylase level is within normal limits.

☐ **4.21** A 23-year-old woman presents with right iliac fossa pain for 4 days, associated with nausea but no vomiting. A dipstick urine test is normal and a careful history reveals offensive vaginal discharge.

THEME: UPPER ABDOMINAL PAIN

Options

A   Bleeding peptic ulcer

B   Biliary colic

C   Cholecystitis

D   Gastric outlet syndrome

E   Lower lobe pneumonia

F   Myocardial infarction

G   Pancreatitis

H   Perforated peptic ulcer

I   Ulcerative colitis

For each of the scenarios described below, select the single most likely diagnosis from the list of options above. Each option may be used once, more than once or not at all.

☐ **4.22** A 33-year-old woman presents with severe abdominal pain radiating to the back. She is shocked and hyperventilating. There is no free gas on her erect chest X-ray. An opacity is noted at the level of the L1 vertebra.

☐ **4.23** A 57-year-old smoker presents with epigastric pain, and sweating, and is vomiting clear fluid. He has a pulse of 58 and a raised jugular venous pressure.

☐ **4.24** A 43-year-old man with multiple sclerosis presents with a pulse of 120 and a rigid abdomen. He is apyrexial. There are no bowel sounds. He has recently completed a course of methylprednisolone.

☐ **4.25** A 47-year-old woman presents with intermittent epigastric pain and vomiting. The pain can last for hours. She has mild epigastric and right upper quadrant tenderness. Bowel sounds are present.

☐ **4.26** An 83-year-old man presents following a collapse. He is not tachycardic but has a postural drop in blood pressure. He has mild epigastric discomfort. You note he has a history of arthritis and hypertension and takes diclofenac and atenolol for these conditions.

THEME: MALABSORPTION

Options

A   Bacterial overgrowth

B   Coeliac disease

C   Dermatitis herpetiformis

D   *Giardia* infestation

E   Intestinal resection

F   Radiation enteritis

G   Tropical sprue

H   Whipple disease

For each of the patients below, choose the single most likely diagnosis from the list of options above. Each option may be used once, more than once or not at all.

☐ **4.27**   A 45-year-old woman presents with tiredness and malaise associated with anaemia. She also has diarrhoea and steatorrhoea. History reveals that she is infertile and had anxiety and depression. She also has osteoporosis.

☐ **4.28**   An 84-year-old woman on long-term omeprazole gives a history of nausea, bloating, steatorrhoea and diarrhoea of 3 months' duration. She is found to have vitamin B_{12} deficiency.

☐ **4.29**   A 38-year-old man presents with a painful abdomen and steatorrhoea along with significant weight loss. He also has cervical lymphadenopathy and small-joint arthropathy.

☐ **4.30**   A 40-year-old businessman recently returned from India presents with diarrhoea, malabsorption and steatorrhoea.

4.31   A 36-year-old man presents with upper abdominal pain. When asked specifically where the pain is, he points to the epigastrium. He says the pain is more during the day and is worse when he is hungry. Antacids relieve it. You suspect he has a duodenal ulcer.

Which one of the following statements about *Helicobacter pylori* is true?

☐ **A**   *Helicobacter* immunoassay on a stool sample can be used for the qualitative detection of the *H. pylori* antigen, and is useful for monitoring the efficacy of eradication therapy

☐ **B**   Histological examination of tissue biopsy samples permits detection of the bacterium without evaluation of tissue damage

☐ **C**   IgG antibodies to *H. pylori* can be found in saliva, and are likely to give false-negative results in those who have recently taken antibiotics, bismuth compounds or omeprazole.

☐ **D**   In infected tissues, it takes about 1 day for the changes in the *Campylobacter*-like organism (CLO) test to become apparent

☐ **E**   The [^{13}C]urea breath test can be used to demonstrate eradication of the organism following treatment

4.32   **Regarding irritable bowel syndrome, which one of the following statements is correct?**

☐ **A**   It is a cause of rectal bleeding
☐ **B**   It is more prevalent in women
☐ **C**   It often has oral symptoms
☐ **D**   It usually presents in childhood
☐ **E**   Weight loss is common

4.33 A 56-year-old-man, who attends surgery infrequently, presents with a 5-week history of heartburn and acid reflux. He returns to see you after a 2-week trial of a proton pump inhibitor (PPI) with partial improvement. His body mass index is 25 kg/m^2.

Which one of the following is the most appropriate next step in his management?

☐ **A** Add an alginate preparation

☐ **B** Continue the PPI and review in 2 weeks

☐ **C** *Helicobacter pylori* testing

☐ **D** Refer for urgent endoscopy

☐ **E** Refer to a dietician for advice including weight loss measures

4.34 A 52-year-old international businessman presents with upper abdominal pain and says he has noticed darker urine. He is overweight.

What is the most likely picture when you check his liver function tests (LFTs)?

A	Bilirubin 120	ALT 170	ALP 946
B	Bilirubin 18	ALT 35	ALP 160
C	Bilirubin 75	ALT 1400	ALP 400

Normal values: bilirubin 3 – 17 μmol/l, alanine aminotransferase (ALT) 5–35 IU/l, alkaline phosphatase (ALP) 30–150 IU/l.

CHAPTER 4 QUESTIONS

ANSWERS

THEME: CAUSES OF CONSTIPATION

4.1   C   Bowel obstruction

Absolute constipation (ie inability to pass flatus as well as faeces) is one of the cardinal features of bowel obstruction. The other features are colicky abdominal pain, distension and vomiting. In small-bowel obstruction, constipation appears after the onset of vomiting; in large-bowel obstruction, vomiting appears later. High-pitched bowel sounds are strongly suggestive of mechanical bowel obstruction. Functional obstruction (pseudo-obstruction) may cause a similar clinical picture but the bowel sounds are often absent.

4.2   A   Anal fissure

Anal fissure is a very common problem and often follows a period of relative constipation. The passage of a hard stool produces a fissure, the pain of which causes anal spasm and further constipation. The resultant vicious cycle can be broken with stool softeners and local anaesthetic preparations. Topical nitrates have also proved useful in reducing spasm. Severe cases may require an anal stretch or lateral sphincterotomy under anaesthesia.

4.3   L   Pregnancy

Pregnancy causes constipation due to the presence of a pelvic mass and reduced gastrointestinal motility. Indigestion occurs later as smooth muscle relaxation reduces the tone of the gastro-oesophageal sphincter and results in acid reflux. Pregnancy in young women may present late, even in the absence of learning difficulties.

4.4   G   Hypercalcaemia

The combination of depression, fatigue, constipation and bone pain is suggestive of hypercalcaemia. In a man of this age, the likely cause is malignant disease. Back pain that prevents the patient sleeping is also suspicious for metastases or myeloma. Hypothyroidism could also explain most of the symptoms but not the back pain. Colorectal carcinoma does not usually produce bone metastases.

4.5   I   Iatrogenic

Patients in hospital often develop constipation for a number of reasons including pain, poor fluid intake, lack of dietary fibre, immobility and medication. It would be unlikely that a routine hysterectomy would result in bowel obstruction directly. However, it is likely that opioid analgesia, given for postoperative pain, will cause constipation if adequate fluids, fibre and/or laxatives are not provided. Nausea may be due to impending bowel obstruction or due directly to the opioids. Pinpoint pupils also suggest the patient is receiving excess opioids.

4.6   E   Carcinoma of the rectum

Tenesmus, the feeling that the bowel is incompletely emptied after evacuation, is a symptom that is associated with rectal tumours (carcinoma or polyps) and irritable bowel syndrome. It is unusual for irritable bowel syndrome to develop in a patient of older age and the presence of anorexia and weight loss is more consistent with cancer.

THEME: CAUSES OF HEPATOMEGALY

4.7   G   Infectious mononucleosis

Glandular fever (infectious mononucleosis) may cause liver or spleen enlargement in about 10% of cases. Occasionally the organs are painful due to rapid expansion causing stretching of the capsule. Rarely, splenic enlargement may be so rapid that the spleen is liable to rupture. Liver function tests are often deranged but rarely done.

4.8   H   Liver metastases

Liver metastases commonly arise from bowel and breast. Palpable metastases need not have any effect on liver function, which is only impaired if the metastases involve over half the liver or if there is biliary obstruction.

4.9   C   Congestive cardiac failure

Right heart failure is often forgotten as a cause of ascites and hepatomegaly, due to congestive changes. In tricuspid regurgitation, the enlarged liver may be pulsatile. The commonest causes of right heart failure are left heart failure, hypertension and valvular disease. Rheumatic fever rarely causes tricuspid or pulmonary valve lesions, so this patient probably has cardiac failure primarily due to aortic or mitral valve disease or hypertension.

CHAPTER 4 ANSWERS

4.10 B Amyloidosis

Patients with chronic inflammatory diseases may develop secondary amyloidosis. Causative conditions include rheumatoid arthritis, bronchiectasis and chronic osteomyelitis. Amyloid accumulates in lymphoreticular and other tissues, such as the tongue and skin. Purpura may be due to cutaneous amyloid or hypersplenism-induced thrombocytopenia. Cardiac amyloid is rare in secondary amyloid. Amyloid also causes nephrotic syndrome. Felty syndrome is the main differential diagnosis in a patient with hepatosplenomegaly and rheumatoid arthritis. However, in this syndrome patients also have lymphadenopathy, neutropenia, anaemia and thrombocytopenia. The main complication is infection.

4.11 I Lymphoma

Patients with lymphoma may either present with a lump (or lumps) or with generalised symptoms. Of particular importance are 'B symptoms' – weight loss, fever, night sweats – which affect the choice of treatment and prognosis of the disease. Involvement of extra-nodal sites, such as liver, spleen and bone marrow, puts this patient at stage 4B. This is the highest stage and carries the worst prognosis. Treatment is chemotherapy after histological confirmation. Lymph node pain on drinking alcohol is said to be a feature of Hodgkin disease.

THEME: CAUSES OF DYSPHAGIA

4.12 J Reflux oesophagitis

Gastro-oesophageal reflux disease (GORD) is associated with smoking, high alcohol intake, hiatus hernia, pregnancy, obesity, systemic sclerosis and tight clothes. Gastric acid enters the oesophagus through the incompetent lower oesophageal sphincter. This results in oesophageal inflammation, which if extensive may result in dysphagia and eventually oesophageal stricture or Barrett oesophagus. Patients may complain of heartburn, an acid taste in the mouth (acid brash), excessive salivation (waterbrash), difficulty in swallowing and nocturnal asthma.

4.13   A   Achalasia

Oesophageal achalasia involves failure of relaxation of the circular muscles at the lower end of the oesophagus associated with loss of the myenteric plexus of nerves in this region. Oesophageal dilatation occurs above the area of achalasia. The condition tends to present between the ages of 30 and 40 years and is slightly more common in women. Dysphagia gradually progresses over years. In addition to regurgitation of partially digested food and halitosis, patients may aspirate on lying flat (hence the coughing) and so are susceptible to aspiration pneumonia. The diagnosis may be obvious on a chest X-ray showing a wide mediastinum and a shadow behind the heart with a fluid level. The diagnosis can be confirmed with a barium swallow or endoscopy. Treatment of severe achalasia is usually surgical (Heller operation) but mild achalasia may respond to nitrates and anticholinergic medication.

4.14   I   Plummer–Vinson syndrome

Plummer–Vinson syndrome or Paterson–Brown–Kelly syndrome consists of iron deficiency anaemia, glossitis, angular cheilitis and dysphagia due to a postcricoid oesophageal web. A friable web lies across the anterior oesophageal lumen and may be seen on endoscopy and a barium meal. It is caused by epithelial hyperplasia and hyperkeratosis of the oesophageal mucosa. The condition is premalignant and the patient should undergo biopsy. The iron deficiency anaemia should be investigated and treated appropriately.

4.15 H Pharyngeal pouch

The development of a pharyngeal pouch is often preceded by a history suggestive of reflux oesophagitis or hiatus hernia. It has been hypothesised that oesophageal hypertrophy occurs in an attempt to prevent acid reflux and that this causes a relative obstruction at the level of cricopharyngeus muscle with the resultant pressure causing protrusion of a mucosal pouch at the level of Killian dehiscence between thyreopharyngeus and cricopharyngeus. This pouch is usually easily demonstrated in the upper neck on a barium swallow. Again patients are prone to aspiration of semi-digested food which leads to episodes of coughing and aspiration pneumonia. Management is surgical with excision of the pouch.

4.16 E Left atrial hypertrophy

The description of the clinical findings suggests that this patient has significant mitral stenosis. The associated large left atrium may favour atrial fibrillation with palpitations and pressure on the oesophagus may result in dysphagia. Radiological features of mitral stenosis associated with enlargement of the left atrium include a double cardiac silhouette, straightening of the left border of the heart and a horizontal left bronchus.

THEME: ACUTE ABDOMEN

4.17 D Leaking aortic aneurysm

A leaking abdominal aortic aneurysm may mimic many other causes of acute abdomen. The classic triad of a pulsatile mass, severe back pain and profound hypotensive collapse has a poor prognosis, and these patients frequently do not make it to hospital alive. The clues here are the age, the sex and the signs of cardiovascular instability.

4.18   G   Perforated peptic ulcer

Non-steroidal anti-inflammatory drugs are widely used, and have a detrimental effect on the kidneys and the gastrointestinal tract. Gas under the diaphragm indicates a perforated viscus and these patients will usually have advanced signs of peritonitis.

4.19   I   Ureteric colic

The pain of ureteric colic is very severe and will often be described as the worst pain a patient has ever experienced. The characteristic restlessness and inability to find a position that is comfortable is highly suggestive of this condition. A dipstick urine test will usually be positive for blood, and a ureteric calculus will sometimes be seen on X-ray.

4.20   E   Mesenteric ischaemia

Mesenteric ischaemia occurs in patients with arteriopathy. Risk factors therefore include an arrhythmia such as atrial fibrillation, advanced age, smoking and diabetes. Postprandial pain and weight loss may denote so-called 'mesenteric angina'. Progression to intestinal gangrene may show as dilated loops of bowel with 'thumb printing' on a plain abdominal X-ray film, and a blood gas assay may show a metabolic acidosis with profound base deficit. It is a diagnosis of exclusion but the pain the patient experiences may be disproportionately severe to the clinical signs.

4.21   A   Acute salpingitis

The false-negative rate for appendicitis is highest in fertile young women and in this group a careful gynaecological history should always be taken, and ultrasound scan and even laparoscopy considered. The history for appendicitis is usually brief, 24–48 hours, and will usually be associated with gastrointestinal symptoms such as anorexia, nausea, vomiting or diarrhoea. A longer history, combined with a vaginal discharge is suggestive of pelvic inflammatory disease, but often this diagnosis is only made at the time of removing a normal appendix.

THEME: UPPER ABDOMINAL PAIN

4.22   G   Pancreatitis

Gallstones are infrequently visible on X-ray but are the commonest cause of acute pancreatitis in the UK. Pancreatitis is also associated with binge drinking or chronic alcohol use, mumps, trauma, and can occur in the postoperative period following upper abdominal surgery. The diagnosis is usually based on the history and very raised serum amylase.

4.23   F   Myocardial infarction

The raised jugular venous pressure indicates right-sided heart failure. Myocardial infarction is an important cause of epigastric pain and an electrocardiogram should always be done.

4.24   H   Perforated peptic ulcer

The assessment of patients with serious and existing disease can be very difficult. This man has recently received methylprednisolone and is at increased risk of upper gastrointestinal bleeding or perforation. The presence of a rigid abdomen and no bowel sounds should always raise the suspicion of bowel perforation. Gas in the peritoneal cavity, shown on an erect chest X-ray or supine lateral abdominal X-ray, is a sign of perforated peptic ulcer disease

4.25   B   Biliary colic

Intermittent epigastric symptoms with a tender right upper quadrant are associated with biliary colic. If accompanied by jaundice, urgent ultrasound scan is required to exclude a gallstone in the common bile duct because of a risk of ascending cholangitis. Acute cholecystitis may occur on a background of biliary colic, but with a presentation including fever, occasionally with rigors, severe right upper quadrant pain and a positive Murphy sign.

4.26   A   Bleeding peptic ulcer

This man is taking non-steroidal anti-inflammatory drugs (NSAIDs) for his arthritis. Gastrointestinal bleeding is a frequent cause of collapse in elderly people. The hypovolaemia is manifested as the postural drop in blood pressure. The patient is not tachycardic because he is taking β-blockers for his hypertension.

THEME: MALABSORPTION

4.27   B   Coeliac disease

Besides the symptoms and signs mentioned in the question, manifestations include tetany, osteomalacia and even gross malnutrition leading to peripheral oedema. Polyneuropathy and paraesthesia may also occur.

4.28   A   Bacterial overgrowth

Excess bacterial growth occurs in the small intestine which normally contains few organisms. Risk factors include the use of medication, such as proton pump inhibitors, and anatomical disturbances of the bowel. The treatment is with antibiotics given in a cyclical manner to prevent bacterial tolerance.

4.29   H   Whipple disease

This is a rare systemic infection caused by the bacterium *Tropheryma whipplei*. The heart, lung, brain, joints and eyes may also be involved. Histologically, the villi are stunted and contain diagnostic PAS-positive macrophages. Treatment is with suitable antibiotics for 1–2 years.

4.30   D   *Giardia* infestation

The causative organism (*Giardia lamblia*) can be found in jejunal fluid or mucosa. It is a flagellate protozoan parasite. Cases are more commonly associated with recent foreign travel.

4.31   E   The [^{13}C]urea breath test can be used to demonstrate eradication of the organism following treatment

Patients infected with *H. pylori* have immunoglobulin antibodies to the organism. Tests for the detection of antibodies to *H. pylori* circulating in the blood, or found in the saliva, have excellent sensitivity and specificity of over 95%, and are cheap and simple compared with invasive techniques. They can give very quick results even within minutes of the first consultation, and are the only tests that are not likely to give false-negative results in patients who have recently taken antibiotics, bismuth compounds or omeprazole (National Institutes of Health Consensus Conference, 1994). Immunoassay in stool can only be used for qualitative detection. Histological examination of tissue biopsy samples (usually four, taken from different parts of the stomach lining) permits detection of the bacterium together with evaluation of tissue damage. Most cases of infection can be detected with a haematoxylin and eosin (H&E) stain of gastric tissue, but special stains like Giemsa can be used if the H&E stain is inconclusive. In infected tissues the change occurs within about an hour, so that the results of the *Campylobacter*-like organism (CLO) test are often available while the patient is still in the endoscopy unit, meaning that decisions about treatment can be made immediately.

4.32   B   More prevalent in women

Irritable bowel syndrome is a common condition that affects women more than men. It usually causes symptoms of altered bowel habit but without red flag symptoms such as rectal bleeding. Abdominal pain is often relieved by defecation. Weight loss is not a symptom, and if present should alert the clinician to other underlying pathology.

4.33   B   Continue the PPI and review in 2 weeks

Take a full history and thoroughly examine patients presenting with new-onset dyspepsia (which can be deduced from this scenario as the patient infrequently attends the surgery). A trial of 1 month PPI is usually suggested, though there is inadequate evidence whether this or *H. pylori* testing should be offered first. People of any age who present with dyspepsia in association with chronic gastrointestinal bleeding, unintentional weight loss, dysphagia, vomiting, epigastric mass or iron deficiency anaemia should be referred for urgent endoscopy (as per NICE guidelines 2004 (www.nice.org.uk/cgo17).) Also, in those patients over 55 years of age with persistent unexplained dyspepsia (ie 4–6 week history with no obvious cause), urgent endoscopy should also be requested.

4.34

A	Bilirubin 120	ALT 170	ALP 946

This man has presented with cholestatic jaundice, and the pain suggests gallbladder disease as an aetiology, most likely gallstones. The LFTs would show raised bilirubin with marked rise in ALP compared with transaminases. Albumin level would be normal. Approximately 70% of causes of cholestatic jaundice are extrahepatic. This man would need an ultrasound scan to assess his liver and biliary tree.

CHAPTER 4 ANSWERS

Chapter 5
Infectious diseases, Haematology, Immunology and Genetics

QUESTIONS

THEME: INTERPRETATION OF HAEMATOLOGICAL RESULTS

Options

A   β-Thalassaemia minor

B   Acute myeloid leukaemia

C   Alcoholic liver disease

D B_{12} deficiency

E   Chronic lymphocytic leukaemia

F   Chronic myeloid leukaemia

G   Cytotoxic drugs

H   Folate deficiency

I   Iron deficiency

J   Myelodysplasia

K   Old age

L   Rheumatoid arthritis

For each set of results below, choose the single most likely diagnosis from the above list of options. Each option may be used once, more than once or not at all.

Normal values

- White cell count (WCC): 4.0–11.0 x 10^9/l

- Neutrophils: 2.0–7.5 x 10^9/l

- Lymphocytes: 1.3–3.5 x 10^9/l

- Monocytes: 0.2–0.8 x 10^9/l

- Haemoglobin (Hb): men 13.5–18.0 g/dl; women 11.5–16.0 g/dl

- Red cell count: men 4.5–6.5 x 10^{12}/l; women 3.9–5.6 x 10^{12}/l

- Mean corpuscular volume (MCV): 76–97 fl

- Mean corpuscular haemoglobin (MCH): 27–32 pg

- Platelet count: 150–400 x 10^9/l

- Ferritin: 12–200 µg/l

☐ **5.1** **40-year-old woman: Hb 9.0 g/dl, MCV 82 fl, WCC 8.1 x 10^9/l, platelets 450 x 10^9/l, serum ferritin 300 mg/l.**

☐ **5.2** **50-year-old man with longstanding epilepsy: Hb 10.1 g/dl, MCV 115 fl, WCC 3.8 x 10^9/l (lymphocytes 2.5, neutrophils 1.3), platelets 243 x 10^9/l.**

☐ **5.3** **21-year-old woman, booking visit to antenatal clinic: Hb 9.7 g/dl, MCV 71 fl, MCH 27 pg, red cell count 6.7 x 10^{12}/l, WCC 6.4 x 10^9/l, platelets 310 x 10^9/l, HbA2 5%.**

☐ **5.4** **75-year-old woman, investigations for fatigue: Hb 9.4 g/dl, MCV 102 fl, WCC 4.5 x 10^9/l (lymphocytes 1.8, neutrophils 1.7, monocytes 1.0, myeloblasts 0.1), platelets 190 x 10^9/l.**

☐ **5.5** **60-year-old man, routine blood test: Hb 10.8 g/dl, MCV 87 fl, MCH 30 pg, WCC 18.4 x 10^9/l, platelets 190 x 10^9/l. Direct antiglobulin test – positive.**

☐ **5.6** **55-year-old man, routine blood test: Hb 13.8 g/dl, MCV 106 fl, WCC 6.7 x 10^9/l, platelets 110 x 10^9/l. Blood film – target cells and hypersegmented neutrophils.**

THEME: ADVICE FOR TRAVELLERS – VACCINATIONS

Options

A   All of E and yellow fever also

B   All of A and meningitis (types A and C) also

C   Hepatitis A vaccine only

D   Hepatitis A, typhoid and polio vaccines

E   Hepatitis A and B, typhoid, polio, diphtheria and rabies vaccines

F   No precautions required

G   Rabies vaccine only

H   Typhoid and polio vaccines only

I   Typhoid vaccine only

For each of the traveller descriptions given below, choose the most appropriate advice from the above list of options. Each option may be used once, more than once or not at all. Assume each patient is currently resident in the UK.

☐ **5.7**   **A doctor is travelling to Somalia to work for the International Red Cross.**

☐ **5.8**   **A businessman going to a conference in Thailand.**

☐ **5.9**   **A 40-year-old man intending to travel to Barbados for a holiday. He had hepatitis A 4 years ago and received polio vaccine as a child.**

☐ **5.10**   **A 12-year-old girl travelling to rural France with her parents.**

THEME: VIRAL INFECTIONS IN CHILDHOOD

Options

A   Adenovirus

B   Cytomegalovirus (CMV)

C   ECHO virus

D   Enterovirus

E   Epstein–Barr virus

F   Mumps

G   Molluscum contagiosum (pox virus)

H   Rotavirus

For each group of symptoms listed below, select the most likely causative agent from the list of options above. Each option may be used once, more than once or not at all.

☐ **5.11**   A 4-month-old child of an human immunodeficiency virus (HIV)-positive mother is perfectly well until he develops a cough and tachypnoea. He soon requires ventilation and the chest X-ray shows bilateral pneumonitis.

☐ **5.12**   A 10-year-old boy develops high fever with generalised lymphadenopathy and hepatosplenomegaly 4 weeks after he has a liver transplant.

☐ **5.13**   An 18-month-old boy from a travelling family is admitted with unilateral parotid swelling and has signs of meningism.

☐ **5.14**   A 3-year-old has a crop of raised discrete lesions with umbilicated centres on his abdomen. They persist for several months but the child remains well.

THEME: VACCINES

Options

A Hib

B Mantoux

C Pneumovax

D Rubella

E Salk polio

F Tetanus

For each description given below, choose the most likely vaccine from the above list. Each option may be used once, more than once or not at all.

☐ **5.15 Killed**

☐ **5.16 Conjugate**

☐ **5.17 Live**

☐ **5.18 Polysaccharide**

THEME: CONGENITAL INFECTIONS IN CHILDHOOD

Options

A Cytomegalovirus infection

B Herpes simplex infection

C Parovirus

D Rubella

E Syphilis

F Toxoplasmosis

In each of the following clinical scenarios, which one of the congenital infections listed above is the most likely? Each option may be used once, more than once or not at all.

☐ **5.19** A newborn baby with thrombocytopenia, hepatosplenomegaly, retinitis and periventricular calcification on computed tomography (CT) of the head.

☐ **5.20** A newborn baby girl with hepatosplenomegaly, chorioretinitis, and tram-like calcifications on CT of the head.

☐ **5.21** A newborn baby boy with skeletal changes suggestive of recurrent periostitis, a bony prominence of the head and a saddle nose.

☐ **5.22** A stillborn child with non-immune (ie compatible rhesus constellation) hydrops fetalis.

THEME: HAEMATOLOGICAL CONDITIONS

Options

A   Acute lymphoblastic leukaemia

B   Acute myeloid leukaemia

C   Acute promyelocytic leukaemia

D   Chronic lymphocytic leukaemia

E   Chronic myeloid leukaemia

F   Hodgkin lymphoma

G   Monoclonal gammopathy of undetermined significance

H   Multiple myeloma

I   Non-Hodgkin lymphoma

J   Waldenström macroglobulinaemia

For each of the following scenarios, choose the most likely diagnosis from the list of options above. Each option may be used once, more than once or not at all.

☐ **5.23**   A 70-year-old retired farmer is found to have a peripheral blood lymphocytosis when a full blood count is done after he presents to his GP with herpes zoster.

☐ **5.24**   A 60-year-old African Caribbean man presents to his GP with persistent bony pains. Initial blood investigations reveal an anaemia, raised erythrocyte sedimentation rate (ESR), urea and creatinine, and hypercalcaemia.

☐ **5.25**   A pale 4-year-old girl with recurrent infections and ophthalmoplegia undergoes a full blood count. A subsequent bone marrow investigation shows primitive pre-B lymphoblast cells.

☐ **5.26**   An HIV-positive man on effective antiretroviral therapy presents with painless lymphadenopathy and fevers, drenching night sweats and weight loss.

☐ **5.27** A pale, thin 50-year-old bank manager presents with tiredness, weight loss and sweating. He has noticed some visual disturbances. Examination reveals splenomegaly. Haematological investigation reveals massive neutrophilia with left shift but low neutrophil alkaline phosphatase score and a high serum vitamin B_{12} level.

THEME: RED BLOOD CELLS

Options

A   Fragment cells

B   Hypochromia, anisocytosis, poikilocytosis

C   Pancytopenia with hypocellular bone marrow

D   Pancytopenia with normal bone marrow function

E   Raised mean corpuscular volume (MCV) with macrocytosis and normal bone marrow

F   Raised MCV with megaloblasts in bone marrow

G   Raised red cell count and bone marrow erythroid hyperplasia

H   Sickle cells

I   Sideroblasts, basophilic stippling

J   Spherocytes and reticulocytes

In each of the following clinical scenarios, which one of the above sets of blood/bone-marrow results would represent the most likely findings. Each option may be used once, more than once or not at all.

☐ **5.28   A 56-year-old man with pernicious anaemia.**

☐ **5.29   A 63-year-old man with a prosthetic heart valve.**

☐ **5.30   A 23-year-old man has previously been admitted for recurrent chest pains and now presents with priapism.**

☐ **5.31   A 45-year-old woman with rheumatoid arthritis and a large spleen.**

☐ **5.32   A 9-year-old boy with lead poisoning.**

☐ **5.33   A 31-year-old Tanzanian man with hookworm infection.**

THEME: SEXUALLY TRANSMITTED DISEASES

Options

A   Candidiasis

B   *Chlamydia trachomatis*

C   Gonorrhoea

D   Herpes simplex virus

E   Human papilloma virus

F   Lymphogranuloma venereum

G   Primary syphilis

H   Secondary syphilis

I   Trichomonal vaginosis

For each of the following clinical scenarios, chose the single most likely diagnosis from the list of options above. Each option may be used once, more than once or not at all.

- [ ] **5.34** A 28-year-old woman has an offensive, profuse, green-grey vaginal discharge. No lesions are visible on speculum examination.

- [ ] **5.35** There is a painless indurated ulcer on the penis of a 35-year-old man. Smear from the ulcer base is positive to dark-field examination.

- [ ] **5.36** Small painless vulval ulcer in a 29-year-old woman who presents with enlarged lymph nodes in the groin. There are sinuses from the matted nodes.

- [ ] **5.37** A 24-year-old woman presents with painful urinary retention. She has clusters of small ulcers on the vulva and around the urethra.

- [ ] **5.38** A 29-year-old man returns from holiday abroad complaining of a milky urethral discharge.

5.39 A 46-year-old HIV-positive man, on treatment, develops fever, malaise and anorexia. He also complained of diarrhoea and is found to have malabsorption and anaemia. The organism responsible is isolated on direct examination and culture of a bone marrow sample. He is being treated with a combination of ethambutol, rifabutin and clarithromycin.

Which of the following organisms is the most likely cause?

- ☐ **A** *Cryptosporidium parvum*
- ☐ **B** *Mycobacterium avium intracellulare*
- ☐ **C** *Mycobacterium tuberculosis*
- ☐ **D** *Pneumocystis jiroveci*
- ☐ **E** *Pseudomonas aeruginosa*

5.40 Which one of the following statements regarding 'Tamiflu' is correct?

- ☐ **A** Its generic name is zanamivir
- ☐ **B** It is taken as a nasal spray
- ☐ **C** It can be used in adults and children aged over 1 year
- ☐ **D** It is licensed only for treatment of influenza

5.41 In genetics, what is the mode of inheritance of red-green colour blindness?

- ☐ **A** Autosomal dominant
- ☐ **B** Autosomal recessive
- ☐ **C** Polygenic inheritance
- ☐ **D** X linked

CHAPTER 5 QUESTIONS

5.42   A 24-year-old woman has had an itchy red rash on her left
wrist for 1 month. She also has red scaly areas on her ear
lobes.

**Which is the single most likely diagnosis from the list
below?**

☐ **A** Allergic urticaria

☐ **B** Atopic eczema

☐ **C** Chrome dermatitis

☐ **D** Nickel dermatitis

☐ **E** Seborrhoeic eczema

ANSWERS

THEME: INTERPRETATION OF HAEMATOLOGICAL RESULTS

5.1   L   Rheumatoid arthritis

Anaemia with a low-normal MCV suggests either partially treated iron deficiency, mixed haematinic deficiency, thalassaemia or anaemia of chronic disease. A high ferritin excludes the first two possibilities. In a 40-year-old woman, chronic disease is the most likely cause and rheumatoid arthritis is a common chronic disease that causes anaemia. A moderately elevated platelet count is also consistent with an inflammatory condition.

5.2   H   Folate deficiency

Macrocytosis, anaemia and neutropenia suggest megaloblastic anaemia, which is caused by deficiency of vitamin B_{12} or folate. Phenytoin impairs folate metabolism and causes actual or functional folate deficiency. Macrocytosis without anaemia is common in patients treated with phenytoin.

5.3   A   β-Thalassaemia minor

Minor thalassaemias (β-or α) cause mild anaemia, with microcytosis out of proportion to the mean cell haemoglobin. They also cause an elevated red cell count, which helps to distinguish them from iron deficiency. HbA2 is formed by 2 α chains and 2 δ chains and is found in low levels (< 3%) in normal individuals. Levels are increased where β-chain production is impaired. The anaemia is rarely of clinical importance except in pregnancy.

5.4   J   Myelodysplasia

Myeloblasts are seen in myeloid leukaemia, leukaemoid reaction, leukoerythroblastic syndromes and myelodysplasia. Myelodysplasia is common in the elderly but is not a feature of normal ageing. Any or all of the cell lines may be reduced. Monocytosis and mild macrocytosis is common and small numbers of myeloblasts may occur. There is no specific treatment, although folate supplements may help. Treatment is symptomatic – transfusion for anaemia, antibiotics for infection, platelet transfusions rarely. The condition may transform into acute myeloid leukaemia.

5.5   E   Chronic lymphocytic leukaemia

Chronic lymphocytic leukaemia is common and is often identified as an incidental finding on blood tests in older people. It may also present with lymphadenopathy, hepatosplenomegaly, bruising, anaemia or recurrent infections. There may be associated thrombocytopenia, anaemia, neutropenia or immunoparesis due to marrow infiltration. Anaemia may also occur due to an associated autoimmune haemolytic anaemia, giving a positive direct antiglobulin (Coombs) test, which may be treated with steroids. Occasionally antiplatelet antibodies also occur.

5.6   C   Alcoholic liver disease

Hypersegmented neutrophils occur in megaloblastic anaemia, uraemia and liver disease. Macrocytosis occurs in megaloblastic anaemia, liver disease, hypothyroidism, myelodysplasia, marrow infiltration, alcohol, pregnancy or haemolysis. Target cells occur in iron deficiency, haemolysis, haemoglobinopathies and liver disease. The common link is liver disease. Alcohol is also directly toxic to platelets.

THEME: ADVICE FOR TRAVELLERS – VACCINATIONS

Any traveller intending to visit a high-risk area should seek expert advice (normally a Practise Nurse gives this advice). Vaccination alone is not enough and travellers should also be advised to use insect nets and sprays and to avoid insect and animal bites. They should also be advised to take condoms (and use them).

5.7   B   All of A and meningitis (types A and C) also

Sub-Saharan Africa has a high level of endemic infections and a broad vaccination programme is recommended. Many countries, but not Somalia, insist on written proof of yellow fever vaccination.

5.8   E   Hepatitis A and B, typhoid, polio, diphtheria and rabies vaccines

Southeast Asia is another high-risk area. Sexually transmitted diseases are common and, apart from hepatitis B, there are no vaccines available as yet.

5.9   H   Typhoid and polio vaccines only

Travellers to the Caribbean are advised to have hepatitis A, typhoid and polio vaccinations. Childhood polio vaccination does not offer lifelong protection; adults are advised to get revaccinated at the same time as their children. Hepatitis A infection probably gives lifelong immunity and so this patient does not need vaccination against it, although it will do him no harm if there is any doubt.

5.10   F   No precautions required

Rabies has been eradicated from the UK but is still present in rural areas of other European countries. The risk is small and rabies vaccine is not given routinely for travel to Western Europe.

CHAPTER 5 ANSWERS

THEME: VIRAL INFECTIONS IN CHILDHOOD

5.11   B   Cytomegalovirus

One has to assume that the child has maternally transmitted HIV and is therefore susceptible to opportunistic infection. Although *Pneumocystis jiroveci* would be the most common cause, CMV infection can prove equally devastating.   (*Pneumocystis jiroveci* is the new name for *Pneumocystis carinii*.)

5.12   E   Epstein–Barr virus

Patients are immunosuppressed following organ transplantation and are especially susceptible to viral infections. This scenario with organomegaly and lymphadenopathy is suggestive of Epstein–Barr-related lymphoproliferative disease, which can affect up to 20% of solid organ recipients.

5.13   F   Mumps

This child is unlikely to have been immunised and is presenting with acute mumps. Meningoencephalitis represents the most severe complication of mumps.

5.14   G   Molluscum contagiosum (pox virus)

The umbilicated centre implies that this is molluscum, a benign condition in childhood although lesions may take months to disappear.

THEME: VACCINES

5.15   **E**   Salk polio

5.16   **A**   Hib

5.17   **D**   Rubella

5.18   **C**   Pneumovax

GP entrants should know the UK vaccination schedule. The full immunisation schedule is give on p. 123. Knowing the nature of the vaccines is also important for giving parents information. At present HIB and meningococcal vaccines are the only conjugate vaccines (a polysaccharide conjugated to a protein carrier) to be used. A simple polysaccharide vaccine in the form of Pneumovax is used for special indications that include post splenectomy and immunosuppressed patients. Measles, mumps and rubella are live attenuated vaccines and although the usual Sabin polio vaccine is a live virus, the killed. Salk vaccine is used for certain patients.

THEME: CONGENITAL INFECTIONS IN CHILDHOOD

5.19   **A**   Cytomegalovirus (CMV) infection

5.20   **F**   Toxoplasmosis

5.21   **E**   Syphilis

5.22   **C**   Parvovirus

Congenital infections in children can be very similar in presentation, especially congenital rubella, toxoplasmosis and CMV. They are best differentiated on the basis of eye involvement and the type of calcifications observed. Congenital syphilis results in chronic inflammation of the bones and a bony prominence of the head. Congenital parvoviral infection must be considered in all cases of non-immune hydrops.

THEME: HAEMATOLOGICAL CONDITIONS

5.23   **D**   Chronic lymphocytic leukaemia

This is the commonest adult leukaemia in the UK, accounting for up to 40% of all leukaemias. The median age of diagnosis is 65–70 years and the male:female ratio is 2:1. It generally follows an indolent course and in the early stages patients are asymptomatic but may have splenomegaly. Lymphadenopathy, anaemia, herpes zoster, bacterial infections, autoimmune haemolysis or thrombocytopenia may cause the presentation.

5.24   **H**   Multiple myeloma

This clinical scenario is suggestive of multiple myeloma, a tumour of bone marrow plasma cells. Bone pain is the commonest presenting feature and is associated with bone destruction and subsequent hypercalcaemia. Plain X-rays may reveal osteoporosis, lytic lesions and evidence of pathological fractures. Renal impairment is common and is usually due to tubular damage caused by Bence Jones proteins. Other causes of renal impairment in myeloma include hypercalcaemia, dehydration, infection, amyloidosis and non-steroidal inflammatory drugs.

5.25   A   Acute lymphoblastic leukaemia

Acute lymphoblastic leukaemias predominantly affect children and may present with clinical features associated with marrow failure, ie anaemia, bleeding and infections. There may also be bone pain, splenomegaly, lymphadenopathy, thymic enlargement and central nervous system (CNS) involvement with cranial nerve palsies as in this case. There is a 60% cure rate with chemotherapy.

5.26   I   Non-Hodgkin lymphoma

Patients with chronic HIV infection are at risk of developing non-Hodgkin lymphoma. As patients with HIV infection live longer, AIDS related malignancies, especially non-Hodgkin's lymphoma are becoming more comon. It is more aggressive than the non-AIDS related lymphoma.

5.27   E   Chronic myeloid leukaemia

This is a clonal disorder of haemopoietic stem cells characterised by the Philadelphia chromosome which is a balanced translocation between chromosomes 9 and 22. It can occur at any age but the median age is 55–60 years with a median survival of 4–5 years. It is a triphasic disease with most patients presenting during the chronic phase which lasts for 2–7 years. In 50% an abrupt transformation into a blast crisis occurs, when treatment becomes ineffective. The other 50% undergo an accelerated phase which then proceeds to blast crisis more gradually. If there is a massive neutrophilia there may be associated visual disturbances, priapism or deafness.

THEME: RED BLOOD CELLS

5.28   F   Raised MCV with megaloblasts in bone marrow

Vitamin B_{12} deficiency causes a megaloblastic anaemia. Vitamin B_{12} is found in animal products but not in plants – it cannot be synthesised by humans. Therefore, both diet and the ability to absorb vitamin B_{12} are factors to consider if deficiency exists. Pernicious anaemia is caused by atrophy of the gastric mucosa with subsequent reduction in production of intrinsic factor, which is required for the absorption of vitamin B_{12} in the ileum.

5.29   A   Fragment cells

These are damaged red blood cells, which have subsequently resealed their cell membrane. They are incomplete and misshapen. Causes include prosthetic heart valves, renal dialysis and microangiopathic haemolytic anaemias.

5.30   H   Sickle cells

Sickle cell patients experience crises which may be spontaneous or initiated by intercurrent infection, cold or hypoxia. Sickling of red blood cells in small vessels may cause severe pain in almost any site. Chest pain and bone pain are common. Priapism is also seen. Patients may also develop severe neurological sequelae and hyposplenism through recurrent splenic infarcts.

5.31   C   Pancytopenia with hypocellular bone marrow

This patient has Felty syndrome – rheumatoid arthritis (RA) with hypersplenism and pancytopenia. Any cause of chronic splenic enlargement may cause hypersplenism with pancytopenia.

5.32   I   Sideroblasts, basophilic stippling

Lead poisoning leads to inhibition of enzymes involved in haem synthesis, causing anaemia. It also inhibits enzymes that disperse excess RNA and results in abnormal staining of red blood cells on a blood film (discrete blue particles – stippling effect).

5.33   B   Hypochromia, anisocytosis, poikilocytosis

This patient has iron deficiency anaemia. This can result from blood loss, poor dietary intake or decreased absorption. Hookworm infestation of the duodenum is the commonest infective cause worldwide.

THEME: SEXUALLY TRANSMITTED DISEASES

5.34   I   Trichomonal vaginosis

This is a common cause of vaginal discharge, caused by the flagellate protozoan, *Trichomonas*. There is a profuse greenish discharge.

5.35   G   Primary syphilis

Primary syphilis presents as a papule in the mucosa of the lower genital tract, mouth or anorectal region. After 1 week it becomes a chancre – a single painless indurated ulcer. Dark-field examination of a smear from the ulcer base demonstrated *Treponema pallidum*.

5.36   F   Lymphogranuloma venereum

Lymphogranuloma venereum is caused by *Chlamydia trachomatis* serotypes L1, L2 and L3. Other serotypes cause a superficial inflammation of the mucosa and are associated with infertility. The classic finding is of matted inguinal lymph nodes with abscess and sinus formation. The primary lesion is a small papule in the lower genital tract which breaks down to form a painless ulcer.

5.37   D   Herpes simplex virus

Herpes simplex is a sexually transmitted disease caused by either herpes simplex virus 1 or 2. The lesions are typical small clusters of vesicles but in the moist environment of the vulva they will often appear as small extremely painful ulcers, which can precipitate urinary retention secondary to pain.

5.38   C   Gonorrhoea

The commonest sexually transmitted disease causing a milky urethral discharge in men is gonorrhoea. Up to 50% of men and women with gonorrhoea are asymptomatic.

5.39   B   *Mycobacterium avium intracellulare* (MAI)

This is typically resistant to standard antituberculous treatments, although ethambutol may be useful. Primary prophylaxis with rifabutin or azithromycin may delay the appearance of MAI, but no corresponding increase in survival has been shown.

5.40   C   It can be used in adults and children aged over 1 year

Tamiflu's generic name is oseltamivir. It is taken orally and should be taken within 48 hours of the onset of flu symptoms. It is a prescription-only medication licensed both for the prevention and treatment of flu in adults and children over 1 year. In practical terms, the National Institute for Health and Clinical Excellence (NICE) has suggested this should be reserved for at-risk groups only when there is a flu outbreak in the community.

5.41   C   X linked

Along with haemophilia and Duchenne muscular dystrophy, red-green colour blindness is X linked and therefore affects males.

5.42   D   Nickel dermatitis

Nickel allergy is very common and once treated the patient needs to avoid nickel jewellery in the future. It produces allergic contact dermatitis with a type IV (cell-mediated or delayed) hypersensitivity reaction.

Full immunisation schedule

When	Vaccine	How
2 months	Diphtheria, tetanus, pertussis (whooping cough), polio and *Haemophilus influenzae* type b (Hib) (DTaP/IPV/Hib)	One injection
	Pneumococcal infection (Pneumococcal conjugate vaccine, PCV)	One injection
3 months	Diphtheria, tetanus, pertussis, polio and *Haemophilus influenzae* type b (Hib) (DTaP/IPV/Hib)	One injection
	Meningitis C (meningococcal group C) (MenC)	One injection
4 months	Diphtheria, tetanus, pertussis, polio and *Haemophilus influenzae* type b (Hib) (DTaP/IPV/Hib)	One injection
	Meningitis C (meningococcal group C) (MenC)	One injection
	Pneumococcal infection (Pneumococcal conjugate vaccine, PCV)	One injection
12 months	*Haemophilus influenza* type b (Hib) and meningitis C (Hib/MenC)	One injection
13 months	Measles, mumps and rubella (German measles) (MMR)	One injection
	Pneumococcal infection (PCV)	One injection
3 years and 4 months to 5 years	Diphtheria, tetanus, pertussis (whooping cough) and polio (dTaP/IPV or DTaP/IPV)	One injection
	Measles, mumps and rubella (MMR)	One injection
13 to 18 years	Diphtheria, tetanus, polio (Td/IPV)	One injection

Source: http://www.immunisation.nhs.uk

Chapter 6
Musculoskeletal

QUESTIONS

THEME: THE PAINFUL KNEE

Options

A Anterior knee pain in a 15-year-old gymnast with no history of trauma

B Giving way and intermittent swelling

C Intermittent locking and swelling in a patient with osteochondritis dissecans

D Pain along the medial joint line, swelling and inability to extend the joint fully

E Pain over the proximal tibia associated with a tender swelling in a young teenager

Match the conditions listed below to the single most likely clinical picture from the list of options above. Each option may be used once, more than once or not at all.

- ☐ **6.1**   **Anterior cruciate ligament rupture**
- ☐ **6.2**   **Loose body**
- ☐ **6.3**   **Chondromalacia patellae**
- ☐ **6.4**   **Medial meniscus tear**
- ☐ **6.5**   **Osgood–Schlatter disease**

THEME: BACK PAIN

Options

A Bony metastasis

B Central disc prolapse

C Dissecting abdominal aortic aneurysm

D L1–L2 disc prolapse

E L4–L5 disc prolapse

F Mechanical back pain

G Osteoporotic vertebral body crush fracture

H Spinal stenosis

I Spinal tuberculosis

For each of the following clinical scenarios, choose the most likely diagnosis from the list of options above. Each option may be used once, more than once or not all.

☐ **6.6** A 33-year-old male company director complains of intermittent lower back pain in the absence of any neurological symptoms or signs. Radiographs are normal.

☐ **6.7** A 43-year-old woman complains of sudden-onset lower back pain radiating down the left leg as far as the heel. She has paraesthesiae over the lateral aspect of the left lower leg and foot. Examination reveals straight leg raising limited to 20° with altered sensation in the above distribution.

☐ **6.8** A 68-year-old woman complains of bilateral buttock and thigh pain associated with back pain after walking 200 m; sitting down relieves the pain. She does not have any symptoms at rest. Examination of the back is unremarkable.

☐ **6.9** A 28-year-old woman has severe lower back pain; she is incontinent of urine. Examination reveals loss of sensation over the perineum and straight leg raise is limited bilaterally.

☐ **6.10** A 72-year-old man complains of severe back pain not responding to rest. He is unable to sleep and has lost 6 kg over the past 2 months. Examination reveals some tenderness in the lumbar region but no neurological abnormalities.

THEME: PAINFUL HIP IN CHILDREN

Options

A Congenital dysplasia of the hip (CDH)

B Irritable hip syndrome

C Osteomyelitis

D Perthes disease

E Septic arthritis

F Slipped upper femoral epiphysis (SUFE)

G Still disease

Match the symptoms and signs listed below with the single most likely condition from the options given above. Each option may be used once, more than once or not at all.

☐ **6.11** A 6-year-old boy complains of intermittent hip pain for several months. Haematological investigations are normal. X-rays show flattening of the femoral head.

☐ **6.12** A 2-year-old girl with a one-day history of increasing hip pain has become unable to weight bear. Her WCC is 22/fl, with an ESR of 88 mm/hour and a CRP of 300 mg/l. A radiograph of the hip shows a widened joint space.

☐ **6.13** A 12-year-old boy with left groin pain for 6 weeks is noticed to stand with the left leg externally rotated. Examination reveals negligible internal rotation of the hip.

☐ **6.14** A 4-year-old boy complains of right hip pain a few days following an upper respiratory tract infection. Blood tests are as follows: wcc 11.0 x 10⁹/l, erythrocyte sedimentation rate (ESR) 10 mm/hour and C-reactive protein (CRP) 2 mg/l.

☐ **6.15** A 5-year-old girl complains of progressively increasing severe pain in her left hip and upper leg for 6 days. She is able to walk but limps visibly. Blood tests are as follows: wcc 19.0×10^9/l, ESR 72 mm/hour and CRP 94 mg/l. X-rays and ultrasound scans of the hip are normal.

THEME: DISORDERS OF THE KNEE JOINT

Options

A Anterior cruciate ligament injury

B Gout

C Meniscal injury

D Osgood–Schlatter disease

E Osteoarthritis

F Osteosarcoma of the proximal tibia

G Patella bursitis

H Patella fracture

I Rheumatoid arthritis

J Septic arthritis

For each of the following patients, select the single most likely diagnosis from the list of options above. Each option may be used once, more than once or not at all.

☐ **6.16** **A 33-year-old nurse was running for the bus when she tripped and fell over an uneven paving slab. She felt something crack and afterwards was unable to bear weight on the leg. In accident and emergency, considerable bruising around the knee is noted. She is unable to lift her leg off the couch.**

☐ **6.17** **A 50-year-old electrician has a tender fluctuant lump that appears to float under the skin of the kneecap. The overlying skin appears normal.**

6.18 A 55-year-old ex-footballer presents to his GP with a long history of aches and pains in various joints. He has had previous meniscectomies of both knees and since he took part in a charity match last weekend he has had considerable pain and swelling in his right knee. He can barely walk. Examination confirms a large tense effusion within the joint and significant restriction in joint movement. He is otherwise well.

6.19 A 55-year-old publican presents to his GP with a 24-hour history of acute pain and swelling in his left knee. He has been unable to sleep. Examination confirmed a large effusion in his knee and considerable tenderness. He is known to have history of recent congestive cardiac failure but no significant musculoskeletal symptoms had been documented previously.

THEME: ACUTE HOT KNEE

Options

A Anterior cruciate ligament disruption

B Baker cyst

C Gonococcal arthritis

D Gout

E Lyme arthritis

F Prepatellar bursitis

G Pseudogout

H Rheumatoid arthritis

I Septic arthritis

J Systemic lupus erythematosus (SLE)

For each of the following clinical scenarios, select the single most appropriate diagnosis from the list of options above. Each option may be used once, more than once or not at all.

☐ **6.20** A 29-year-old woman presents with a swollen knee, pyrexia and an erythematous macular rash on her palms and soles of her feet.

☐ **6.21** A 31-year-old woman presents with a hot swollen knee. Her ESR and CRP levels are raised. She has felt generally unwell for a week.

☐ **6.22** A 67-year-old woman presents with a painful, hot, swollen knee. Her joint aspirate is turbid and shows positively birefringent rhomboid crystals on microscopy.

☐ **6.23** A 12-year-old boy with a hot swollen left knee, raised ESR, pyrexia and severe pain on passive movement. His joint aspirate is turbid.

THEME: RHEUMATOLOGY

Options

A Ankylosing spondylitis

B Gouty arthritis

C Osteoarthritis

D Osteoporosis

E Polymyalgia rheumatica

F Psoriatic arthropathy

G Reiter disease

H Rheumatoid arthritis

I Scleroderma

J Systemic lupus erythematosus

For each of the presentations below, select the single most likely diagnosis from the list of options above. Each option may be used once, more than once or not at all.

☐ **6.24** A 53-year-old woman has swan-neck deformities of her fingers and pain in her hips. X-ray examination reveals erosion of the ends of the phalanges.

☐ **6.25** A 23-year-old African Caribbean woman presents with joint pains. She has a red facial rash. On examination, her hands appear normal.

☐ **6.26** A 56-year-old woman presents with knee and hip pain. X-rays of the hips show narrowing of the joint space and osteophyte formation. Examination of the knees demonstrates marked crepitus.

☐ **6.27** A 25-year-old man presents with a long history of low back pain. He is experiencing the acute onset of heel pain. Examination reveals tenderness beneath the calcaneum and a limited range of spinal movements.

☐ **6.28** An elderly woman complains of shoulder stiffness. She cannot brush her hair or apply her make-up due to the stiffness. She denies true weakness. She attends with acute visual loss in the left eye.

THEME: PAINFUL UPPER LIMB

Options

A Anterior dislocation of the shoulder

B Colles fracture

C de Quervain tenosynovitis

D Fractured surgical neck of humerus

E Gamekeeper's thumb

F Posterior dislocation of the shoulder

G Scaphoid fracture

H Supracondylar fracture of the humerus

I Smith fracture

For each of the scenarios below select the single most likely diagnosis from the list of options above. Each option may be used once, more than once or not at all.

☐ **6.29** A 23-year-old man complains of a painful wrist after falling over while drunk. There is tenderness in the thenar eminence and pain abducting his thumb.

☐ **6.30** A 4-year-old girl presents with a painful swollen arm after falling off a pony. The nurse has difficulty taking the radial pulse.

☐ **6.31** A 35-year-old electrician is brought in with a painful upper limb and chest pain following an accident at work in which he received an electric shock.

☐ **6.32** A 67-year-old woman fell while out shopping. She is clutching her arm to her side and complaining of pain.

☐ **6.33** A 31-year-old factory worker complains of a painful arm, which causes difficulty sleeping. There is swelling on the radial side of her forearm above the wrist, with crepitus felt on movement at this site.

6.34   A 33-year-old married man was visiting Thailand with his family when he developed diarrhoea that lasted for 1 week. He returned to the UK and 2 weeks later presented to his GP complaining of pain in his knee and both heels. His eyes are red and he has developed some painless, red, confluent plaques on his hands and feet, which his GP has diagnosed as psoriasis.

Which one of the following is the most likely diagnosis?

☐ **A**   Ankylosing spondylitis
☐ **B**   Enteropathic arthritis
☐ **C**   Gonococcal arthritis
☐ **D**   Psoriatic arthritis
☐ **E,**   Reactive arthritis

6.35   A 52-year-old man with rheumatoid arthritis does not respond to sulfasalazine and methotrexate and cannot tolerate gold.

Select from the list below the single most appropriate disease-modifying drug that you can use.

☐ **A**   Celecoxib
☐ **B**   Intra-articular corticosteroids
☐ **C.**   Infliximab
☐ **D**   Naproxen
☐ **E**   Oral corticosteroids

6.36 Which of the following is not a 'red flag' sign in a patient with acute back pain?

☐ **A** Absent ankle jerk

☐ **B** Age < 20 years

☐ **C** Pain not exacerbated on movement

☐ **D** Taking steroids

☐ **E** Weight loss

6.37 A 12-year-old boy has a limp and painful heel that is locally tender when squeezed. He is a keen soccer player.

Which one of the following is the most likely diagnosis?

☐ **A** Morton metatarsalgia

☐ **B** Navicular osteochondritis

☐ **C** Pes planus

☐ **D** Plantar fasciitis

☐ **E** Sever disease

ANSWERS

THEME: THE PAINFUL KNEE

6.1   **B**   **Giving way and intermittent swelling**

The anterior cruciate ligament prevents forward subluxation of the tibia on the femur under normal conditions; its rupture results in instability that is usually associated with a joint effusion.

6.2   **C**   **Intermittent locking and swelling in a patient with osteochondritis dissecans**

Loose bodies most commonly arise in knees of patients with osteochondritis dissecans. In this condition there is necrosis of the subchondral bone with subsequent detachment of a fragment of bone and its overlying cartilage. It most commonly affects the lateral surface of the medial femoral condyle.

6.3   **A**   **Anterior knee pain in a 15-year-old gymnast with no history of trauma**

Atraumatic anterior knee pain in a teenager is almost invariably due to chondromalacia. More commonly found in girls who exercise regularly.

6.4   **D**   **Pain along the medial joint line, swelling and inability to extend the joint fully**

A bucket handle meniscal tear can cause locking (ie inability to fully extend the joint). Medial joint pain suggests a medial meniscus problem.

6.5 **E** **Pain over the proximal tibia associated with a tender swelling in a young teenager**

In this condition, there is traction osteochondritis of the tibial tuberosity at the insertion of the patellar tendon. It tends to occur in active boys and is characterised by anterior knee pain and tender swelling of the tibial tuberosity.

THEME: BACK PAIN

6.6 **F** **Mechanical back pain**

A sedentary lifestyle is the usual cause of mechanical back pain. The absence of any neurological abnormalities is necessary for the diagnosis. Physiotherapy with back-strengthening exercises and postural advice is the mainstay of treatment. Weight loss may be advised if needed and keeping active is important for the recovery process.

6.7 **E** **L4–L5 disc prolapse**

This woman has sciatica. The distribution of her leg symptoms suggests compression of the L5 nerve root which is usually caused by an L4–L5 disc prolapse.

6.8 **H** **Spinal stenosis**

Spinal stenosis causes claudication. The symptoms subside within minutes of sitting down. Assessment of the peripheral circulation is mandatory to exclude any vascular causes. Surgical treatment is by spinal decompression.

6.9   B   Central disc prolapse

This is an emergency. Urgent decompression is required to prevent any irreversible damage. The diagnosis is central disc prolapse.

6.10   A   Bony metastasis

Intractable back pain (ie persisting at rest) in an elderly person is unusual. It suggests a malignant process, particularly if associated with systemic symptoms such as weight loss. Spinal tuberculosis is rare in the UK.

THEME: PAINFUL HIP IN CHILDREN

6.11   D   Perthes disease

Perthes disease commonly presents in the 4–9 years age group. It is more common in boys, and often there is a strong family history. The symptoms tend to be relatively minor in the early stages. At a later stage, X-rays may show flattening of the femoral head caused by localised osteonecrosis.

6.12   E   Septic arthritis

This girl has septic arthritis; this condition is characterised by severe pain usually rapid in onset and the child is unable to walk. It occurs most commonly below the age of four years. The commonest organism isolated is *Staphylococcus. aureus*. High inflammatory markers, along with fluid in the hip joint, suggest the diagnosis that is confirmed with joint aspiration. The basis of treatment is surgical drainage with adjuvant antibiotic therapy.

6.13   F   Slipped upper femoral epiphysis (SUFE)

Slipped upper femoral epiphysis is found in older children (boys > girls), up to the age of puberty. Classically, the symptoms are insidious in onset, as the displacement is gradual. External rotation of the limb at rest is pathognomonic. A special lateral X-ray view will show the posterior displacement of the upper femoral epiphysis.

6.14   B   Irritable hip syndrome

Irritable hip may follows an upper respiratory tract infection. The pathophysiology is still unknown. The child develops a form of reactive synovitis in the hip with pain and a sterile effusion. Blood tests are usually normal and children are not systemically ill. Aspiration of the hip joint will reveal fluid containing white blood cells but no organisms. Aspiration is also therapeutic as it reduces pain. Recovery usually occurs in 7–10 days without treatment.

6.15   C   Osteomyelitis

Osteomyelitis can be difficult to differentiate clinically from septic arthritis. The pain tends to be more chronic in onset and less severe. In osteomyelitis the child may still be able to walk, which is not the case with septic arthritis.

THEME: DISORDERS OF THE KNEE JOINT

6.16   H   Patella fracture

A patella fracture occurs when the quadriceps contracts against resistance (in this case when the foot was caught against the paving slab). A crack is often heard when the bone breaks. If the extensor mechanism is effectively ruptured (either by rupture of the quadriceps or patella tendons or by fracture of the patella) the person cannot actively extend the knee or lift the straight leg.

6.17   G   Patellar bursitis

Prepatellar bursitis (housemaid's knee) is the inflammation of the pre-patellar bursa, which lies in front of the patella. The normal function of the bursa is to reduce the friction between the patellar tendon and overlying skin when bending the knee. Acute bursitis can be triggered by injury or infection. Chronic bursitis is a longer term problem. Repeated damage to the knee for example from kneeling or work that involves a lot of pressure on the kneecap, as in this case with an electrician, thickens the walls of the bursa causing irritation.

6.18   E   Osteoarthritis

Primary osteoarthritis is often responsible for widespread aches and pains, whilst secondary osteoarthritis is often more specific to joints which have been damaged previously (for example following meniscectomy). Relatively minor trauma (such as playing a game of football) may lead to an acute exacerbation of symptoms and a joint effusion that understandably is uncomfortable and restricts movement.

6.19   B   Gout

An acutely swollen and painful knee could be a septic joint but in this case the history of heart disease and his profession should make you wonder about his urate levels. (Some diuretics raise blood urate levels as can alcohol!)

THEME: ACUTE HOT KNEE

6.20　C　Gonococcal arthritis

This is a form of septic arthritis, although at the time of presentation the joint fluid may be sterile – *Neisseria gonorrhoeae* may still be cultured from the genital tract. Usually the patient has recovered from the initial pyrexial phase and characteristic rash affecting the palms and soles prior to the onset of the large-joint mono/polyarticular arthritis. Treatment involves ciprofloxacin or tetracyclines.

6.21　H　Rheumatoid arthritis

This woman has a monoarticular swelling secondary to underlying systemic disease. Commonly the small joints of the hand are the worst affected but a monoarticular presentation in a large joint may occur. In rheumatoid arthritis both ESR and CRP are raised during active disease. In systemic lupus erythematosus only the ESR is raised.

6.22　G　Pseudogout

This represents an acute synovitis initiated by calcium pyrophosphate crystal deposition in the joint. It often affects elderly women and is very painful. In younger people it may be associated with underlying pathology – Wilson disease, hyperparathyroidism or haemochromatosis. The crystals seen from the joint aspirate in gout (sodium urate) are negatively birefringent under polarised light.

6.23   I   Septic arthritis

Staphylococcus aureus is the commonest cause of septic arthritis. In children *Haemophilus influenzae* must also be considered. Occasionally, other Gram-negative organisms may be involved. The infected joint is hot, swollen and very painful, and usually held in a fixed position as a result of spasm in the surrounding muscles. The patient is usually pyrexial and blood cultures are often positive. Joint aspirate is turbid and should be sent for microscopy and culture. A joint washout and systemic antibiotics are required.

THEME: RHEUMATOLOGY

6.24   H   Rheumatoid arthritis

Rheumatoid arthritis is more common in women than men. Swan-neck deformity and boutonnière deformity of the fingers are characteristic of the condition as is ulnar deviation of the fingers at the metacarpophalangeal joints. The distal interphalangeal joints are usually spared. Radiologically, erosions are the characteristic bone change, along with joint-space narrowing and osteoporosis. Bone destruction is a late finding.

6.25   J   Systemic lupus erythematosus

Systemic lupus erythematosus is nine times more common in women than men. It begins in young adulthood and is more common in those of African and Polynesian descent. The classic rash is a butterfly erythematous facial rash. Joint pain is commonly a prominent feature although examination is usually normal. Serum antinuclear antibodies are positive in almost all cases. Double-stranded DNA antibodies are specific but are seen in only 50% of cases.

6.26   C   Osteoarthritis

Osteoarthritis is a degenerative arthritis affecting the large joints of the lower limbs in particular. The hand and finger joints (especially the distal interphalangeal joints) may be affected, including the carpometacarpal joint of the thumb. Crepitus is a common finding and is usually painless. Radiologically there is narrowing of the joint space and characteristic osteophyte formation.

6.27   A   Ankylosing spondylitis

Ankylosing spondylitis is a condition that becomes clinically apparent in late adolescence to early adulthood. It is more common in men than women. Susceptibility is related to HLA-B27 type. Radiologically, an early sign is erosion and sclerosis of the sacroiliac joints, accounting for the back pain.

6.28   E   Polymyalgia rheumatica

Polymyalgia rheumatica occurs in patients over 60 years of age, predominantly women. It presents with shoulder girdle pain, stiffness, and only occasionally any weakness. Polymyositis presents with proximal muscle weakness. Polymyalgia rheumatica is associated with temporal arteritis, which may result in sudden visual loss. Treatment in this case is urgent high-dose steroids to relieve symptoms and prevent blindness in the other eye.

THEME: PAINFUL UPPER LIMB

6.29   G   Scaphoid fracture

With a scaphoid fracture there is pain on abducting the thumb. The tenderness is in the anatomical snuffbox area (bordered by the tendons of extensor pollicis longus on the ulnar side and extensor pollicis brevis and abductor pollicis brevis on the radial side) as well as in the thenar eminence. Gamekeeper's thumb is disruption of the ulnar collateral ligament of the thumb at the metacarpophalangeal joint with tenderness at this level.

6.30   H   Supracondylar fracture of the humerus

This is an orthopaedic emergency. In a fracture of the supracondylar region of the humerus the triceps pulls the forearm posteriorly, resulting in impingement of the brachial artery on the fracture end. The resultant pressure puts the vascular supply to the forearm at risk, hence the poor

6.31   F   Posterior dislocation of the shoulder

Electric shock and epilepsy are two of the commonest associations with posterior dislocation of the shoulder.

6.32   D   Fractured surgical neck of humerus

In older patients a fracture of the shaft of the humerus is possible and can be associated with radial nerve palsy due to injury to the nerve as it passes down the spiral groove. Falls in women of this age may also result in a Colles fracture of the forearm.

6.33   C   de Quervain tenosynovitis

de Quervain's tenosynovitis occurs as a result of repetitive movements such as may be encountered in factory work. Pain is often worse at night. The swelling is of the sheath around the abductor pollicis longus and extensor pollicis brevis tendons at the radial styloid.

6.34   E   Reactive arthritis

A variety of organisms can trigger reactive arthritis. It is typically an acute, asymmetrical, lower limb arthritis, occurring a few days to a couple of weeks after infection. Sacroiliitis and spondylitis may develop. Acute anterior uveitis may complicate more severe disease. The skin lesions resemble psoriasis (circinate balanitis and keratoderma blenorrhagica). The classical triad of Reiter disease is urethritis, arthritis and conjunctivitis.

6.35   C   Infliximab

Infliximab is a monoclonal antibody directed against tumour necrosis factor-alpha and is given intravenously. Infliximab can be co-prescribed with methotrexate to prevent loss of efficacy because of antibody formation. Both products halt bone erosion in up to 70% of patients with rheumatoid arthritis, with healing in a few. As a side-effect, some people become autoantibody positive and develop a reversible lupus-like syndrome. Reactivation of old tuberculosis may occur.

6.36   A   Absent ankle jerk

Absent ankle reflex is classed as a localised neurological sign and may occur in the first 4 weeks of an acute episode of low back pain without being a red flag sign. Simple musculoskeletal back pain is rare in the under 20 age group and should be investigated for underlying cause. Steroids predispose to loss of bone density and crush fractures. Weight loss and non-mechanical pain suggest malignancy.

6.37   E   Sever disease

Sever disease is osteochondritis in the calcaneal epiphysis and typically occurs in children over 8 years. Osteochondritis causes softening and deformity of bone. It can occur in many sites. A rare site in younger children is the navicular bone. Plantar fasciitis causes inferior heel pain in adults. Pes planus is flat feet and common in young children but is generally painless. Morton metatarsalgia is a cause of foot pain in adults caused by entrapment of the interdigital nerve between the metatarsal heads.

Chapter 7
Paediatrics

QUESTIONS

THEME: CHILDREN WITH COUGHS

Options

A Acute epiglottitis

B Angio-oedema

C Asthma

D Bronchiolitis

E Cystic fibrosis

F Diphtheria

G Foreign-body inhalation

H Pertussis

I Retropharyngeal abscess

J Viral croup

For each of the patients below, choose the single most appropriate diagnosis from the list of options above. Each option may be used once, more than once or not at all.

☐ **7.1** A 2-year-old boy with a history of fever and running nose for 2 days is brought to the surgery in the evening with a barking cough and stridor.

☐ **7.2** A 3-year-old child with a history of raised temperature and coryza for the last 2–3 days develops a paroxysmal spasmodic cough which terminates with a noisy inspiratory sound.

☐ **7.3** A 6-month-old baby is brought to the surgery with dry cough, difficulty in feeding and breathlessness. On examination his chest is hyperinflated, with fine crackles.

☐ **7.4** A 5-year-old girl presents with a sore throat, difficulty in breathing, fever and drooling of saliva. The child is sitting upright, with her mouth wide open.

☐ **7.5** A 6-year-old boy presents with a troublesome nocturnal cough. He gets breathless after sports and his brother suffers from eczema.

☐ **7.6** A 3-year-old child is brought back to see you because of recurrent chest infections and poor weight gain in spite of voracious appetite. On examination he has nasal polyps.

THEME: ABDOMINAL PAIN

Options

A Abdominal migraine

B Acute appendicitis

C Constipation

D Diabetic ketoacidosis

E Hirschsprung's disease

F Infantile colic

G Intussusception

H Irritable bowel syndrome

I Mesenteric adenitis

J Pancreatitis

K Peritonitis

L Renal calculus

M Torsion of the testis

For each of the patients below, choose the single most appropriate diagnosis from the list of options above. Each option may be used once, more than once or not at all.

☐ **7.7** A 3-month-old baby girl is brought in with paroxysmal crying in the evenings. During the paroxysms she draws up her legs.

☐ **7.8** A 5-year-old boy, with a history of cough and swollen neck glands, presents with abdominal pain. On examination his abdomen is soft, but there is no guarding, and he has tenderness in the right iliac fossa.

☐ **7.9** A 2-year-old boy is brought with a sudden-onset colicky pain. He looks pale, draws up his legs during a pain episode and passes a red, jelly-like stool.

☐ **7.10** A 4-year-old boy with anorexia, vomiting and a high temperature presents with abdominal pain that initially is central, and then moves to the right iliac fossa.

☐ **7.11** A 7-year-old boy presents with paroxysmal abdominal pain with facial pallor; he is otherwise well. There is a family history of migraine.

☐ **7.12** An 8-year-old boy complains that he has had intermittent colicky abdominal pain and bloated feeling for months. The pain is relieved by defecation; sometimes his stools are normal and sometimes he is constipated.

THEME: DIARRHOEA

Options

A   Coeliac disease

B   Crohn disease

C   Irritable bowel syndrome

D   Milk intolerance

E   *Salmonella* gastroenteritis

F   Toddler diarrhoea

G   Ulcerative colitis

H   Viral gastroenteritis

For each of the patients below, choose the single most appropriate diagnosis from the list of options above. Each option may be used once, more than once or not at all.

☐ **7.13**   **An 18-month-old child is brought in irritable, with persistent diarrhoea, abdominal distension and wasting of the buttocks.**

☐ **7.14**   **A 4-year-old boy presents with altered bowel motions and stools containing undigested vegetables. Otherwise the child is well and thriving.**

☐ **7.15**   **A 14-year-old girl presents with intermittent fever, diarrhoea and joint pain. On examination she has ulcers in her mouth. Her periods have not yet started and she has poor breast development.**

☐ **7.16**   **A 2-month-old baby, just started being bottle fed, presents with protracted diarrhoea and poor weight gain. She also has eczema.**

THEME: DEVELOPMENTAL MILESTONES OF CHILDREN

Options

A   6 weeks

B   6 months

C   1 year

D   2 years

E   3 years

F   5 years

From the list of options above select the age at which you would expect a normal child to achieve the developmental stages listed below. Each option may be used once, more than once or not at all.

☐ **7.17**   **Sitting unaided**

☐ **7.18**   **Smiling**

☐ **7.19**   **Walks up stairs**

☐ **7.20**   **Dry by day**

☐ **7.21**   **Cruising around furniture**

THEME: FITS AND FAINTS IN CHILDREN

Options

A   Benign paroxysmal vertigo

B   Breath-holding attacks (cyanotic spells)

C   Complex partial seizure

D   Congenital heart block

E   Myoclonic seizure

F   Petit mal

G   Reflex anoxic seizure (pallid spells)

H   Supraventricular tachycardia

I   Syncope

For each patient below, choose the single most likely diagnosis from the list of options above. Each option may be used once, more than once or not at all.

☐ **7.22**   A 10-year-old had three episodes of loss of consciousness, the first two at school and the last on a shopping outing at a crowded summer sale. She was well prior to the attacks (all having occurred when she had been standing among a crowd). She had felt dizzy, nauseated and become pale and sweaty before losing consciousness for about 2 minutes. There was no incontinence but twitching of the fingers was noted. On recovery she felt tired.

☐ **7.23**   A 3-year-old had three episodes of vomiting and sudden onset of ataxia over the past 6 months. The attacks were rather short (5–10 minutes) but during them he appeared frightened and pale and had to lie down. After the attack he was back to normal. It was mentioned that he keeps his eyes down or closed when travelling by car or in a lift.

☐ **7.24** A 15-month-old girl has had recurrent episodes of loss of consciousness precipitated by temper tantrums. She is developmentally within normal limits. When upset she starts with a shrill cry, goes blue and floppy, losing consciousness for about 1 minute during which a few jerky movement of limbs may occur.

☐ **7.25** A 7-year-old boy has had four episodes of loss of consciousness over the past 6 months. Two occurred in the morning soon after he woke up when he was noticed to be in a 'dreamlike state' with his head turned to the right and doing 'pill rolling' movements with his hand. This was followed by loss of posture and a generalised seizure lasting 3–4 minutes.

☐ **7.26** A 3-year-old has a history of five attacks of loss of consciousness associated with minor trauma such as knocking of his head or injury to his finger. He becomes pale, loses consciousness and goes floppy, sometimes twitching slightly. During one attack he had a heart rate of 30 beats per minute which rapidly recovered. He regained consciousness rapidly each time.

THEME: JAUNDICE IN CHILDHOOD

Options

A   ABO incompatibility

B   Biliary atresia

C   Breast milk jaundice

D   Congenital toxoplasmosis

E   Crigler–Najjar syndrome

F   Galactosaemia

G   Gilbert syndrome

H   Glucose 6-phospho-diesterase deficiency

I   Hereditary spherocytosis

For each of the following clinical scenarios, select the correct cause from the list of options above. Each option may be used once, more than once or not at all.

- [ ] **7.27** A newborn develops an unconjugated hyperbilirubinaemia 12 hours after birth associated with a severe metabolic acidosis.

- [ ] **7.28** A baby is jaundiced at birth and on examination has a distended abdomen with organomegaly. The newborn also has convulsions.

- [ ] **7.29** A newborn develops a progressive conjugated hyperbilirubinaemia with pale stools and dark urine.

- [ ] **7.30** A full-term baby develops jaundice on day three, which continues for two weeks. The bilirubin is unconjugated, there is no derangement of other liver function tests and the child remains clinically well.

7.31   A 5-year-old child is brought by his parents. They are worried that he wets his bed every night. A urine culture is normal and the urine is negative for glucose and protein.

Which one of the following would be the most appropriate management option for this child?

☐ **A**   Desmopressin nasal spray

☐ **B**   Oral imipramine

☐ **C**   Prophylactic antibiotics

☐ **D**   Reassure the parents that it will settle with time

☐ **E**   Referral to the specialist for ultrasound and micturating cystourogram

7.32   Which one of the scenarios described below would be most likely to lead to a suspicion of non-accidental injury?

☐ **A**   Blue discoloration of the back of a child

☐ **B**   Mid-clavicular fracture in a 10-day-old child

☐ **C**   Multiple bruises of various age on the shin of a 5-year-old boy

☐ **D**   Torn fraenum in a 4-month-old baby

☐ **E**   Widespread petechial rash in a 2-year-old child

7.33   A week old neonate presents with vomiting and weight loss, floppiness and circulatory collapse. His penis is enlarged and the scrotum pigmented. Blood testing reveals low sodium and high potassium levels. There is a metabolic acidosis and the baby is hypoglycaemic.

Which one of the following is the most likely diagnosis?

- [ ] **A**   Addisonian crisis
- [ ] **B.**   Congenital adrenal hyperplasia
- [ ] **C**   Conn syndrome
- [ ] **D**   Cushing syndrome
- [ ] **E**   Thyrotoxicosis crisis

7.34   Which one of the pubertal changes given below does not normally occur during the age range suggested?

- [ ] **A**   Age of maximal growth spurt (girls): 12 years
- [ ] **B**   Menarche (girls): 11–15 years
- [ ] **C**   Pubic hair development (girls): 10–14 years
- [ ] **D.**   The start of breast development (girls): 12–15 years
- [ ] **E**   Age of maximal growth spurt (boys): 14 years
- [ ] **F**   Development of penis (boys): 10–16 years
- [ ] **G**   Pubic hair growth (boys): 11–16 years
- [ ] **H**   Testicular enlargement (boys): 9–15 years

ANSWERS

THEME: CHILDREN WITH COUGHS

7.1   J   Viral croup

Viral croup is most often caused by the parainfluenza virus. It commonly occurs in children from 6 months to 6 years of age. Typical features are a barking cough, harsh stridor and hoarseness, usually preceded by fever and coryza. Most cases settle without any intervention, but some children need treatment (oral/nebulised dexamethasone) or occasionally admission for partial airways obstruction. Parents should be warned that the stridor can worsen at night, and they should seek help urgently if they feel the breathing is deteriorating.

7.2   H   Pertussis

Pertussis is a highly infectious form of bronchitis caused by *Bordetella pertussis*. After 2–3 days of coryza, the child develops a characteristic paroxysmal or spasmodic cough followed by an inspiratory whoop (which gives pertussis its common name 'whooping cough'). The cough is worse at night and may be followed by vomiting. Epistaxis and subconjunctival haemorrhage may occur. Symptoms persist for 10–12 weeks. Vaccination or infection do not confer lifelong immunity, but are thought to make subsequent infection less severe.

7.3   D   Bronchiolitis

Bronchiolitis is the commonest serious respiratory infection of infancy. Caused by the respiratory syncytial virus in 80% of cases, it is common in the winter months. Coryzal symptoms precede a dry cough and increasing breathlessness. Wheeze is often present. Feeding difficulty is often associated with dyspnoea. There is no specific treatment and management is supportive.

7.4   A   Acute epiglottitis

Acute epiglottitis is a life-threatening emergency because of the respiratory obstruction. It is caused by *Haemophilus influenzae* type B. The disease occurs in children between the ages of 1 and 6 years. Its onset is often very acute, with a high fever and a toxic-looking child. An intensely painful throat stops the child from speaking and swallowing, and saliva drools down the chin. Soft stridor is present. The child sits immobile and upright with an open mouth to optimise their airway. This is a paediatric emergency.

7.5   C   Asthma

Asthma affects 10–15% of schoolchildren. In childhood it is twice as common in boys as in girls, but by adolescence the ratio is equal. Diagnosis is clinical and depends on a history of recurrent wheeze, cough and breathlessness. In pre-school children the main symptom may be a troublesome cough at night. The diagnosis is supported by a history of a triggering factor or of a personal or family history of atopy.

7.6   E   Cystic fibrosis

Cystic fibrosis is inherited as an autosomal recessive disease. In Caucasians, the carrier rate is 1 in 25. Most children present with malabsorption and failure to thrive from birth, accompanied by recurrent chest infections. Finger clubbing is a feature of established disease. Other features are sinusitis, nasal polyps and rectal prolapse. Older children and adolescents may have diabetes mellitus, cirrhosis or pneumothorax, and boys may be sterile.

THEME: ABDOMINAL PAIN

7.7   F   Infantile colic

Infantile colic is common in the first few months of life. Paroxysmal uncontrollable crying withdrawing up of the knees, takes place several times a day, particularly in the evening. The condition resolves by 4 months of age. Advice about how to manage the symptoms is helpful.

7.8   I   Mesenteric adenitis

The associated pain usually resolves within 24–48 hours. It is less severe than appendicitis and tenderness in the right iliac fossa is variable. The disease is most commonly caused by a viral (adenovirus, EBV, Coxsakie B, influenza B) or streptococcal upper respiratory infection. Enteric pathogens such as Sampylobacter, Salmonella or Yersina can also be responsible.

7.9   G   Intussusception

Intussusception occurs between 2 months and 2 years of age. It is caused by invagination of the proximal bowel into the distal segment. No underlying intestinal cause is found. A viral illness causing enlargement of Peyer patches may stimulate the lead point. Presenting features are a severe paroxysmal colicky pain and pallor – the child becomes pale, especially around the mouth, and draws their legs up during episodes of pain. A sausage-shaped mass is often palpable in the abdomen. Passage of a stool containing blood-stained mucus, abdominal distension and shock should be treated with immediate resuscitation and reduction.

7.10   B   Acute appendicitis

This is the commonest cause of abdominal pain in childhood requiring surgical intervention. Common symptoms are anorexia, vomiting and abdominal pain that is initially central but then localises to the right iliac fossa. Signs are a flushed face with bad breath, fever, tenderness and guarding at McBurney point. Perforation is common in children as the omentum is less developed and fails to surround the appendix.

7.11   A   Abdominal migraine

Abdominal pain usually accompanies cranial migraine, but in children the abdominal pain may be the predominant feature. The pain is usually midline, paroxysmal, with facial pallor. Usually, there is a personal or family history of migraine. Pizotifen can be a helpful prophylactic agent in children with frequent symptoms (to be used under specialist guidance).

7.12   H   Irritable bowel syndrome

This syndrome is associated with altered gastrointestinal motility. There is a positive family history and it is associated with anxiety and stress. Symptoms are bloating, a mucous stool, a feeling of incomplete defecation, constipation alternating with a loose stool, and the relief of pain by defecation.

THEME: DIARRHOEA

7.13   A   Coeliac disease

Coeliac disease is an enteropathy in which gluten provokes a damaging immunological response in the proximal small intestinal mucosa. It commonly presents in the first 2 years of life following the introduction of gluten in cereals. General irritability, abnormal stools, abdominal distension and wasting of the buttocks are common symptoms. In late childhood, children present with anaemia, growth failure and non-gastrointestinal symptoms. Diagnosis is by jejunal biopsy which reveals a flat mucosa (resolves with gluten withdrawal). Anti-endomysial antibody is useful for screening.

7.14   F   Toddler diarrhoea

Toddler diarrhoea is the commonest cause of persistent loose stools in pre-school children. The stool may sometimes be well formed, sometimes explosive and loose. The presence of undigested vegetable in the stool gives it the alternative name of 'peas and carrot syndrome'. The child is usually well and thriving, with no precipitating dietary factor. The condition usually settles by the time the child is 5 years old. Usually no treatment is required. Occasionally, loperamide is given (cautiously).

7.15   B   Crohn disease

Crohn disease is a chronic inflammatory disease affecting any part of the gastrointestinal tract from mouth to anus, but commonly affecting the distal ileum and proximal colon. The affected intestine is thickened, with histological examination showing non-caseating epithelial-cell granulomas. Common features are diarrhoea, abdominal pain, growth failure and puberty delay. Oral and perianal ulcers, anal fistulas, skin tags and fissures are common. Other features are arthritis, uveitis and erythema nodosum. Treatment involves suppression of inflammation by steroids, azathioprine maintains remission. Complications such as fissure, fistula, obstruction and growth failure require surgery.

7.16   D   Milk intolerance

This is common in infants with IgA deficiency and a family history of atopy. It usually manifests as diarrhoea, vomiting, failure to thrive, migraine and eczema, and occasionally with urticaria, stridor and shock. Jejunal biopsy will show a patchy enteropathy with prominent eosinophils in the lamina propria. Most children outgrow their intolerance by 2 years of age. Avoidance of the offending antigen leads to resolution of symptoms. Soya milk is often given but 30% of children are intolerant to soya and hydrolysate-based formula is preferred.

THEME: DEVELOPMENTAL MILESTONES OF CHILDREN

7.17   **B**   6 months

7.18   **A**   6 weeks

7.19   **D**   2 years

7.20   **E**   3 years

7.21   **C**   1 year

In chronological order most normal children smile at 6 weeks, sit at 6 months, cruise around furniture at 1 year, walk upstairs by 2 years and are dry by day at approximately 3 years. All these stages have ranges but in the question only one normal age has been given for each milestone, eg cruising around furniture is delayed at 3 years and incredibly precocious at 6 months so one year is the only possible answer. Major developmental milestones at 6, 12, 18, 24, 36 and 48 months should be learnt. These can be divided into gross motor, fine motor, hearing and language, and social skills.

THEME: FITS AND FAINTS IN CHILDREN

7.22   I   Syncope

Simple syncope results from transient fall in blood pressure due to vasovagal stimulation (dysautonomia syncope) by a variety of stimuli such as pain, fear and standing for a long time, especially in a warm environment. There is a prodrome of dizziness, nausea, buzzing sensation in ears, pallor, sweating and loss of tone followed by loss of consciousness. The electroencephalogram (EEG) does not show epileptic discharges during the episode.

7.23   A   Benign paroxysmal vertigo

This child has typical features of benign paroxysmal vertigo. There is no loss of consciousness, the main feature being transient ataxia. During an attack horizontal nystagmus may be noted. There is increased tendency to have motion sickness.

7.24   B   Breath-holding attacks

This child has typical breath-holding attacks that are precipitated by her being upset and angry. Expiration and apnoea, leading to cyanosis and loss of consciousness, follow the initial cry. The child is bradycardic and may exhibit a few jerky movements. These are self-limiting or respond to behavioural interventions, and cause no lasting damage.

7.25   C   Complex partial seizure

This child has complex partial seizures. There seems to be an aura and some lateralisation at the onset of the seizure that subsequently becomes generalised.

CHAPTER 7 ANSWERS

7.26   G   Reflex anoxic seizure

Reflex anoxic syncope first appears around 1 year of age and is precipitated by sudden pain or fright. The child stops breathing and rapidly loses consciousness, becoming hypotonic and pale. There may be a tonic seizure. There is marked bradycardia or a short period of asystole. Recovery is spontaneous and rarely requires intervention.

THEME: JAUNDICE IN CHILDHOOD

7.27   A   ABO incompatibility

Jaundice within the first 24 hours of life is pathological, and often due to haemolysis. As rhesus incompatibility is preventable ABO incompatibility is now the commonest cause in the UK.

7.28   D   Congenital toxoplasmosis

These signs are suggestive of a congenital infection. Congenital toxoplasmosis results in hepatosplenomegaly, thrombocytopenia and cerebral calcifications. The baby also has convulsions.

7.29   B   Biliary atresia

Biliary atresia is a congenital defect in which there are variable degrees of abnormality of the biliary tract resulting in a progressive obstructive jaundice. Surgical intervention is invariably necessary.

7.30   C   Breast milk jaundice

This scenario is highly suggestive of breast milk jaundice especially since liver function tests and the clinical condition are normal. It is caused by hormonal interaction (5-β-pregnane-3-α-20 β-diol) of breast milk with hepatic enzymes, and will go away if left untreated. The bilirubin is mainly unconjugated, and no kernicterus has been reported with this kind of jaundice.

7.31   D   Reassure the parents that it will settle with time

About 15% of children have enuresis at the age of 5 years: 5% of 10-year-olds and 1% of 15-year-olds still wet the bed. The boy:girl ratio is 2:1. Treatment is not undertaken until a child is 6 years of age. In this case, both the child and parents should be given an explanation and reassurance. Star charts and an enuresis alarm are effective in motivated children. Desmopressin tablets, can be prescribed for children over 7 years of age for short-term intervention (eg school trips or combined with other measures as part of training) but *BNFC* guidance should be followed. Intranasal demopressin is no longer recommended because it has a greater risk of hyponatraemia, water intoxication and convulsions. Imipramine is avoided due to its side-effects and the risk of overdose.

7.32   D   Torn fraenum in a 4-month-old baby

A mid-clavicular fracture in a 10-day-old baby is most likely to be the result of a difficult delivery and a history of the mode of birth should be taken. Although a facial petechial rash may be a sign of smothering, it could be due to a cough, as in whooping cough. A generalised petechial rash should raise the suspicion of idiopathic thrombocytopenic purpura or meningococcal septicaemia. A blue discoloration on the back of an infant is Mongolian blur spot. It is a harmless congenital blue marking on the buttock or sacrum and is commonly mistaken for abuse. Bruises, of different ages, in a 5-year-old child is a normal finding, but it would be suspicious if the child was less than 7 months of age. Common signs of suspicious non-accidental injury are bite marks, a torn fraenum from forced bottle feeding, ligature marks, and burns and scalds.

7.33   B   Congenital adrenal hyperplasia

Congenital adrenal hyperplasia is a rare condition (incidence of approximately 1 in 5000 births) caused by a deficiency of adrenal enzymes. There is autosomal recessive inheritance, and it is more common in consanguineous relationships and certain ethnic populations (eg Ashkenazi Jews or Eskimos). About 90% of cases are due to deficiency of 21-hydroxylase, involved in cortisol production, and up to 80% of cases have impaired aldosterone synthesis. Accumulation of androgenic precursors can cause virilisation and ambiguous genitalia, which means affected females may be mistaken for males at birth. These children need lifelong steroid replacement therapy and if the condition is not detected early they can become severely unwell due to salt wasting from lack of aldosterone.

7.34   D   The start of breast development (girls): 12–15 years

Breast development typically starts at 8–12 years of age. This is usually the first sign of pubertal development in a girl and starts before menarche and pubic hair development.

Chapter 8
Pharmacology and Therapeutics

QUESTIONS

THEME: TERATOGENIC DRUGS

Options

A   Combined oral contraceptive

B   Diethylstilbestrol

C   Digoxin

D   Lithium

E   Phenytoin

F   Progestogens

G   Propylthiouracil

H   Tetracycline

I   Thalidomide

J   Warfarin

For each of the adverse effects described below, choose the single most likely maternal medication taken during pregnancy from the list of options above. Each option may be used once, more than once or not at all.

☐ 8.1   **Children may have discoloured teeth.**

☐ 8.2   **A high dose of this drug is associated with clear-cell vaginal adenocarcinoma and urogenital abnormality in the child.**

☐ 8.3   **Babies born with a small head size and hypoplastic nose.**

☐ 8.4   **Babies born to mothers taking this medication can have neural tube defects, hypoplastic nails and a cleft palate.**

☐ 8.5   **Babies born with short limbs and/or missing limbs.**

THEME: OVER-THE-COUNTER (OTC) MEDICATIONS

Options

A   1% hydrocortisone ointment

B   Chlorphenamine

C   Esomeprazole

D   Ferrous sulphate

E   Loperamide

F   Loratadine

G   Malathion lotion

H   Paracetamol

I   Should be investigated first

J   Sodium alginate

K   Sodium cromoglycate nasal spray

L   Topical clotrimazole

M   Xylometazoline nasal spray

For each of the patients below, choose the single most appropriate medication from the list of options above. Each option may be used once, more than once or not at all.

☐ **8.6**   A 24-year-old woman complains of vulval itching and a white vaginal discharge.

☐ **8.7**   A 30-year-old man complains of heartburn and indigestion, which is worse on lying down.

☐ **8.8**   A 3-year-old girl is febrile and irritable with a generalised vesicular rash. She has a history of a febrile convulsion in the past.

☐ **8.9** A 21-year-old student has hay fever. He is due to take his final exams and is worried that the hay fever will affect his performance. However, he is also worried that medication may make him drowsy.

☐ **8.10** A 56-year-old man has a 2-month history of epigastric pain after meals. His recent blood results reveal iron deficiency anaemia.

THEME: CHOICE OF CONTRACEPTION

Options

A   Barrier methods

B   Combined oral contraceptive

C   Intrauterine contraceptive device

D   Laparoscopic sterilisation

E   Post-coital high-dose levonorgestrel

F   Progesterone depot injection

G   Progesterone-only pill

H   Rhythm methods

I   Vasectomy

For each of the clinical scenarios below, choose the single most appropriate management from the list of options above. Each option may be used once, more than once or not at all.

☐ **8.11**   A couple both aged 38 have three children and request a reliable form of contraception. The wife is concerned about the risks of the combined oral contraceptive. They are very sure they do not want any more children.

☐ **8.12**   A 25-year-old shift worker wishes to avoid pregnancy for at least the next 6 months. She has regular classic migraines. Her partner has latex allergy.

☐ **8.13**   A 35-year-old married woman has two children and would like reliable contraception. She is not absolutely sure that she and her husband will not want a third child at some stage. She smokes 10 cigarettes a day.

☐ **8.14**   A 21-year-old woman had unprotected intercourse at a party 2 days ago. She does not wish to become pregnant.

☐ **8.15**   A 28-year-old woman has discovered that her partner has been using intravenous heroin. She wishes to continue having a sexual relationship with him.

THEME: SIDE-EFFECTS OF DRUGS

Options

A Amiodarone

B Aspirin

C Atenolol

D Carbimazole

E Chlorpromazine

F Erythromycin

G L-Dopa

H Lisinopril

I Lithium

J Metformin

K Sulfasalazine

L Verapamil

For each group of side-effects below, choose the most likely causative agent from the list of options above. Each option may be used once, more than once or not at all.

☐ **8.16** Cold hands and feet, fatigue, impotence

☐ **8.17** Peripheral neuropathy, pulmonary fibrosis, hyperthyroidism

☐ **8.18** Postural hypotension, involuntary movements, nausea, discoloration of the urine

☐ **8.19** Thirst, polyuria, tremor, rashes, hypothyroidism

☐ **8.20** Sore throat, rash, pruritus, nausea

THEME: WARNINGS FOR SPECIFIC DRUGS

Options

A Avoid exposure of the skin to direct sunlight

B May cause blue-tinted vision

C May reduce effect of contraceptive

D Must avoid alcoholic drinks

E Must be taken on an empty stomach

F Must be taken with food

G Not to be stopped without doctor's advice

H Not to be taken with antacids

I Not to be taken with iron tablets

J Take with a full glass of water at least 30 minutes before breakfast and remain upright until after breakfast

For each of the drugs below, choose the single best advice from the list of options above. Each option may be used once, more than once or not at all.

☐ **8.21** **Metronidazole**

☐ **8.22** **Ferrous sulphate**

☐ **8.23** **Prednisolone**

☐ **8.24** **Alendronate**

☐ **8.25** **Amoxicillin**

THEME: DRUGS IN CHILDHOOD

Options

A Aminophylline
B Aspirin
C Azithromycin
D Benzylpenicillin
E Cefotaxime
F Griseofulvin
G Ibuprofen
H Isoniazid
I Terbinafine
J Tetracyclines

For each of the clinical scenarios below, select the correct drug from the list of options above. Each option may be used once, more than once or not at all.

☐ **8.26** Is recommended as first-line empirical intravenous treatment in bacterial meningitis where the cause of infection is not known.

☐ **8.27** Is not recommended for analgesic or antipyretic use in children under 12 years of age due.

☐ **8.28** This is the only licensed systemic agent for dermatophyte skin infection in children under 12 years.

☐ **8.29** Should not be given to children under 12 years of age as it can cause staining and malformation of teeth.

THEME: DRUG INTERACTIONS

Options

A Amoxicillin

B Bumetanide

C Cefalexin

D Cimetidine

E Ciprofloxacin

F Minocycline

G Protamine sulphate

H Spironolactone

I Streptokinase

J Vitamin K

From the list above select the drug most likely to be responsible for the adverse event described in the following case scenarios. Each option may be used once, more than once or not at all.

☐ **8.30** A 57-year-old patient with chronic asthma, who is taking theophylline, is being treated for dysuria and frequency by her GP. She is brought into the emergency department with a pulseless ventricular tachycardia.

☐ **8.31** A 61-year-old man with a prosthetic heart valve is taking warfarin. In hospital for an angiogram, his international normalised ratio (INR) is noted to be 6.9 and he has a severe nosebleed. The house officer starts treatment without consulting his senior colleagues. Twelve hours later the patient has a new cardiac murmur and severe heart failure.

☐ **8.32** A 43-year-old man is taking ciclosporin following renal transplantation. He is treated for a 'chest infection'. Three days later, after admission to hospital, he is noted to have severe renal failure.

8.33 A 67-year-old man, who is taking digoxin for atrial fibrillation, is brought into the emergency department with severe muscular weakness. There are multiple ventricular ectopic beats and small T waves on the electrocardiogram (ECG).

8.34 A 64-year-old with non-insulin-dependent diabetes usually well controlled with metformin and diet is brought into the emergency department unconscious. On testing, his bedside glucose reading (BM stix) is 2.0. He has recently started a new medicine prescribed by his GP.

8.35   A 26-year-old obese man presents to the clinic. His body mass index (BMI) is 36 kg/m^2 and he wants advice regarding treatment of his obesity. He is dieting and has lost 3 kg in weight in the first 4 weeks but is finding it difficult and weight loss has stopped.

Which one of the following would be the single most useful drug to prescribe?

- [ ] **A** Fenfluramine
- [ ] **B** Fluoxetine
- [ ] **C** Levothyroxine
- [ ] **D** Methyl cellulose
- [ ] **E** Orlistat

8.36   Which one of the following drugs does not interact with warfarin?

- [ ] **A** Cimetidine
- [ ] **B** Ibuprofen
- [ ] **C** Metronidazole
- [ ] **D** St John's Wort
- [ ] **E** Vitamin B$_{12}$

8.37   A 27-year-old professional man, presently stable on 20 mg fluoxetine for mild depression, is seeking advice about resuming driving his car.

Which one recommendation by the DVLA applies in this case?

- [ ] **A** A licence is usually refused
- [ ] **B** He can resume driving if there is no other complication
- [ ] **C** He should refrain from driving for 6 months
- [ ] **D** He should refrain from driving for 12 months
- [ ] **E** He should refrain from driving pending a medical report

ANSWERS

THEME: TERATOGENIC DRUGS

8.1   H   Tetracycline

Tetracycline is deposited in teeth and in growing bone as it binds to calcium, and can cause dental staining and growth defects, and altered bone growth. Tetracyclines are contraindicated in pregnant or breastfeeding women and in children under 12 years.

8.2   B   Diethylstilbestrol

Diethylstilbestrol, when given in large doses to pregnant women in the first trimester, has been associated with clear-cell adenocarcinoma of the vagina, an increased risk of infertility and urogenital abnormalities in their daughters and hypospadias in their sons.

8.3   J   Warfarin

Warfarin crosses the placenta and if taken during the first trimester of pregnancy can cause a hypoplastic nasal bridge and chondrodysplasia. During the third trimester warfarin leads to an increased risk of placental or fetal haemorrhage.

8.4   E   Phenytoin

This antiepileptic drug is associated with an increased risk of neural tube defects, cleft lip and cleft palate. Women who become pregnant while taking phenytoin should be carefully monitored and should take folic acid supplements.

8.5   I   Thalidomide

Thalidomide, which was used in the 1950s to treat morning sickness in pregnant women, causes disruption and cessation of limb formation in the fetus (phocomelia). The drug was banned in the early 1960s. In the late 1990s it was re-introduced for the treatment of erythema nodosum leprosum in leprosy and the management of some patients with acquired immune deficiency syndrome (AIDS)/human immunodeficiency virus (HIV) infection and myeloma. The mechanism of phocomelia is still unknown and there are strict guidelines governing the use of thalidomide in women of childbearing age.

THEME: OVER-THE-COUNTER (OTC) MEDICATIONS

8.6   L   Topical clotrimazole

Thrush may be treated with topical clotrimazole cream or a pessary. Other topical antifungal imidazoles are also available over the counter. Oral fluconazole is also available without prescription. Topical clotrimazole is cheaper bought over the counter than with a prescription.

8.7   J   Sodium alginate

Upper gastrointestinal symptoms in a young man are usually due to benign pathology. National Institute for Health and Clinical Excellence (NICE) guidance (2004) (www.nice.org.uk/cg017) indicates that in the absence of alarm signs, dyspepsia thought to be due to gastro-oesophageal reflux disease (GORD) should be treated with a course of a cost-effective proton pump inhibitor (eg omeprazole, which is now available over the counter) or 'test and treat' for *Helicobacter pylori*. This can be combined with simple lifestyle measures and alginate preparations (eg Gaviscon) or other OTC medications at the lowest dose that control symptoms. Lifestyle advice includes weight loss, smoking cessation, avoiding alcohol and other drugs associated with dyspepsia (eg non-steroidal anti-inflammatory drugs (NSAIDs)), eating earlier in the evening, and propping up the head end of the bed if possible. Esomeprazole is not available over the counter.

8.8   H   Paracetamol

The diagnosis is a viral illness, possibly chickenpox. There is no specific treatment indicated for uncomplicated chickenpox. The most important action is to bring down her temperature to reduce the risk of a second febrile convulsion. Parents should be advised to keep the child in a cool room with minimal clothing, to sponge the child with tepid water and to use a fan. Paracetamol is useful as an antipyretic and also an analgesic. Aspirin is not recommended because of the risk of Reye's syndrome. If itch is a major problem, topical calamine lotion or an oral antihistamine may be used. Several antihistamines are licensed for use in children, including loratadine, promethazine and chlorphenamine, for allergic conditions but not pruritus. Only one antihistamine, azatadine, is licensed for use for pruritus.

8.9   F   Loratadine

Several antihistamines are licensed for use for seasonal or perennial allergic rhinitis. Loratadine is a non-sedating antihistamine. Chlorphenamine is sedating and should be avoided if a patient needs to maintain concentration. An alternative for the student would be to use topical sodium cromoglicate. However, a nasal spray alone will not be sufficient, as allergic conjunctivitis is likely to be equally problematic.

8.10   I   Should be investigated first

NICE guidance states that patients with dyspepsia plus any alarm signs (chronic gastrointestinal bleeding, progressive unintentional weight loss, progressive difficulty swallowing, persistent vomiting, iron deficiency anaemia, epigastric mass, or suspicious barium meal) or an unexplained recent-onset persistent dyspepsia in a person aged 55 years or over should prompt urgent referral for endoscopy.

THEME: CHOICE OF CONTRACEPTION

8.11   I   Vasectomy

The most effective form of contraception is sterilisation of either the male or female partner. If they are quite sure that they do not want more children then this would be the management of choice. Vasectomy is preferable to female sterilisation as it does not require a general anaesthetic and the complication rate is lower. If there is any doubt, an intrauterine contraceptive device provides good protection with minimal inconvenience. Oestrogen-containing contraception is associated with increased thrombotic complications in older women.

8.12   F   Progesterone depot injection

The combined oral contraceptive is contraindicated in women with migraine, and although the progesterone-only pill could be used, it is not as effective in someone this age who is likely to have good fertility. Long-acting reversible methods of contraception would be ideal in this situation, as she does not wish to become pregnant for at least the next 6 months. The intrauterine contraceptive device would be an option here, but can be technically difficult in nulliparous women. The ideal option is the depot progesterone injection, as this confers reliable contraception for 3 months, and does not rely on scrupulous compliance by the patient, as with most forms of progesterone-only pills.

8.13   C   Intrauterine contraceptive device

This is probably the best form of contraception for an older woman in a stable relationship, and has a similar failure rate to sterilisation.

8.14 E Post-coital high-dose levonorgestrel

Post-coital contraception aims to prevent implantation in case of fertilisation. One option is high-dose levonorgestrel (either with or without oestradiol) within 72 hours of unprotected intercourse. The other option is insertion of an intrauterine contraceptive device within 5 days. In a young woman, levonorgestrel is the treatment of choice. Vomiting is a common side-effect, particularly if it is given with oestradiol. The woman should be warned that if she does vomit, she would need to have the tablets re-prescribed. An antiemetic is often prescribed in addition (not metoclopramide because of the risk of extrapyramidal side-effects in young women).

8.15 A Barrier methods

Barrier methods will protect her against sexually transmitted viruses (HIV, hepatitis B and C, herpes) as well as pregnancy.

THEME: SIDE-EFFECTS OF DRUGS

8.16 C Atenolol

Use of β-blockers is often limited by their side-effects. Fatigue and impotence, in particular, are commonly described. In fact, impotence is a potential side-effect of most antihypertensives, including angiotensin-converting enzyme (ACE) inhibitors, thiazide diuretics and some calcium channel blockers (eg nifedipine and amlodipine). It is quite likely that, in many cases, the main cause for erectile dysfunction is the hypertension and not the drug.

8.17   A   Amiodarone

Amiodarone can cause many adverse effects, which limits the use of this otherwise versatile antiarrhythmic. It may affect many organs:

- Lungs: alveolitis, fibrosis, pneumonitis
- Thyroid: hyperthyroidism, hypothyroidism (both common)
- Liver: jaundice, hepatitis, cirrhosis, raised transaminases
- Nervous system: nightmares, neuropathy, headache, ataxia, tremor
- Musculoskeletal: myopathy, arthralgia
- Eyes: reversible corneal microdeposits, optic neuritis (rare)
- Skin: photosensitivity, dermatitis, persistent slate-grey discoloration (rare)
- Heart: bradycardia, conduction disturbances

8.18   G   L-Dopa

L-Dopa-containing drugs often cause gastrointestinal disturbance, particularly nausea, which may be minimised by taking the tablets on a full stomach. Urine and other body fluids may be stained red. Cardiovascular effects include postural hypotension, which may limit the dose that the patient will tolerate (severe postural hypotension should raise the possibility of multisystem atrophy as a cause of parkinsonism and autonomic failure). Neurological side-effects may occur early (dizziness, agitation and insomnia) or late (dyskinesias, psychosis and hallucinosis). Dyskinesias may occur with peak L-dopa levels or with 'wearing-off'.

8.19   I   Lithium

Thirst, polyuria, fine tremor and weight gain are common side-effects of lithium. Lithium may induce nephrogenic diabetes insipidus after prolonged usage. Patients may develop goitre with lithium and some will go on to become hypothyroid. Lithium is reabsorbed in the kidney by the same mechanism as sodium and water. Patients may develop lithium toxicity if they become dehydrated or hyponatraemic. Early lithium toxicity causes coarse tremor, agitation and twitching. Later features are coma, convulsions, arrhythmias and renal failure. Treatment is supportive with hydration and anti-convulsants as required. Dialysis is occasionally needed in severe cases.

8.20   D   Carbimazole

Nausea and gastrointestinal upset are common, non-specific side-effects of carbimazole. Rashes and pruritus are also quite common and are allergic in origin. A patient who develops a rash should be switched to propylthiouracil. Agranulocytosis and neutropenia is a rare idiosyncratic reaction to carbimazole. Patients should be specifically counselled to report any sign of infection immediately, especially a sore throat, and an urgent full blood count should be done. Agranulocytosis is reversible on stopping the drug.

THEME: WARNINGS FOR SPECIFIC DRUGS

8.21   D   Must avoid alcoholic drinks

Metronidazole inhibits aldehyde dehydrogenase and causes acetaldehyde to accumulate in the blood. A disulphiram-like reaction occurs and patients may complain of facial flushing, throbbing headache and palpitations. A patient taking metronidazole orally should abstain from drinking alcohol while taking the drug and for 48 hours after stopping.

8.22   H   Not to be taken with antacids

Iron is best absorbed in the presence of vitamin C, but inhibited by milky drinks or tannins in tea. Antacids inhibit the absorption of most medications, due to chelation by calcium. This is particularly the case with tetracycline antibiotics, which bind to calcium in the body (this is how they stain teeth). Patients should be advised to avoid taking antacids or other calcium supplements at the same time of day as other medication.

8.23   G   Not to be stopped without doctor's advice

Prolonged use of prednisolone depresses the ability of the body's adrenal glands to produce corticosteroids. Abruptly stopping can cause symptoms of corticosteroid insufficiency, with nausea, vomiting and possible shock. Therefore, withdrawal of prednisolone is usually gradual, which also reduces the risk of an abrupt flare of the disease under treatment

8.24   J   Take with a full glass of water at least 30 minutes before breakfast and remain upright until after breakfast

Alendronate is associated with a risk of oesophageal spasm, pain, ulcers and strictures. Patients may reduce this risk by following the advice given in the question. This certainly limits compliance with an otherwise useful drug. Patients should also be warned to stop the drug and seek medical attention if they develop oesophageal symptoms.

8.25   C   May reduce effect of contraceptive

Amoxicillin and other broad-spectrum antibiotics may cause reduced oral contraceptive efficacy. This is due to the loss of bowel flora that normally recycle ethinyloestradiol from the large bowel. The risk is relatively small but patients should use barrier methods during the course of antibiotics and for a week afterwards. Rifampicin, on the other hand, is a potent hepatic enzyme inducer and almost certainly renders standard dose contraceptives useless.

THEME: DRUGS IN CHILDHOOD

8.26   E   Cefotaxime

Cefotaxime is now recommended by both UK and US academic panels as the drug of choice for empirical treatment in bacterial meningitis. Ceftriaxone is an alternative. In younger age groups, amoxicillin should be added to cover against *Listeria* infection. If parenteral treatment is needed in the community, some local protocols still recommend benzyl penicillin.

8.27   B   Aspirin

This is due to the risk of Reye's syndrome. Reye's syndrome is fatty necrosis of the liver that can lead to fulminant liver failure and encephalopathy and is thought to be caused by certain drugs, especially aspirin.

8.28   F   Griseofulvin

There is a particular need for systemic antifungal treatment in tinea capitis. Although terbinafine is a more effective drug it is not licensed for use in children, but many doctors do use it. Griseofulvin is licensed but finding a suitable preparation for children can be problematic as it is only easily available in tablet form. Tinea capitis is a dermatophyte infection. Dermatophyte infections elsewhere in children can be treated differently.

8.29   J   Tetracyclines

Tetracyclines have long been associated with the staining and malformation of teeth and are not recommended for younger children. They can also cause photosensitivity and can be teratogenic.

THEME: DRUG INTERACTIONS

8.30   E   Ciprofloxacin

Ciprofloxacin increases the plasma levels of theophylline, leading to an increased risk of cardiac arrhythmias. If the two drugs are to be used together, the theophylline dose should be reduced and the plasma theophylline levels closely monitored.

8.31   J   Vitamin K

The house officer has presumably given vitamin K. A symptomatic patient with a high INR and a prosthetic heart valve should have a controlled reduction of the INR. If the INR drops below the required therapeutic level the patient is at risk of clots forming on the prosthetic valve, leading to valve failure and embolic phenomena. Reduction of the INR in these patients should be discussed with the haematology department.

8.32   E   Ciprofloxacin

Ciclosporin is a calcineurin inhibitor. It is may be used to suppress the immune system and has a major role in post-transplant immunosuppression to prevent and treat graft-versus-host disease. It is also markedly nephrotoxic and requires drug level monitoring to ensure a therapeutic range is achieved. Drugs such as quinolones (ciprofloxacin), vancomycin, co-trimoxazole and aminoglycosides increase the risk of ciclosporin toxicity. Macrolides directly increase plasma ciclosporin levels.

8.33   B   Bumetanide

Digoxin toxicity may produce cardiac arrhythmias or heart block. Hypokalaemia caused by a potent loop diuretic may predispose a patient to digoxin toxicity. Correction of the electrolyte disturbance and withdrawal of digoxin will usually correct the situation. For those with life-threatening digoxin overdose, specific digoxin antibodies may be given.

8.34   D   Cimetidine

Cimetidine inhibits the renal elimination of metformin, leading to higher plasma levels. This in turn may lead to hypoglycaemia.

8.35   E   Orlistat

Orlistat inhibits pancreatic lipase, an enzyme that breaks down triglycerides in the intestine. Without this, triglycerides from the diet are prevented from being hydrolysed into absorbable free fatty acids and are excreted undigested. NICE guidance (www.nice.org.uk/cg43) suggests that the drug can be prescribed for adults who after dietary, exercise and behavioural approaches have been started and evaluated have not reached their target weight or have reached a plateau.

- have lost at least 2.5 kg by dieting
- increased activity in the month prior to their first prescription
- have a BMI of 28 kg/m^2 or more and have another serious illness which persists despite standard treatment (eg type 2 diabetes, high blood pressure and/or high cholesterol) or a BMI of 30 kg/m^2 or more with no associated illnesses.

8.36   E   Vitamin B$_{12}$

Warfarin acts as a vitamin K antagonist as its structure is similar. Vitamin K will displace warfarin from its position blocking the production of prothrombin, returning the clotting cascade to normal in 6–12 hours in high enough doses. Warfarin is metabolised in the liver by cytochrome P450 enzyme to inactive 7-hydroxywarfarin. Drugs which induce CP450 will speed up warfarin inactivation so antagonise its effect (eg St John's Wort). Drugs which inhibit hepatic enzymes will decrease warfarin inactivation so potentiate its effect (eg metronidazole, cimetidine). Ibuprofen is a substrate of the same P450 enzyme as warfarin, so may displace it, slow down its metabolism and enhance its effect. Vitamin B$_{12}$ has no part in the clotting cascade and does not affect liver enzymes.

8.37   B   He can resume driving if there is no other complication

A person with uncomplicated depression or anxiety who is stable on treatment can return to driving, providing there is no complication from the medication prescribed, eg medications with a sedative side-effect. Fluoxetine is not a sedative antidepressant. In severe depression or severe anxiety the DVLA should be informed and driving stopped, pending medical recommendation (a period of stability is required before driving can be resumed). In mild dementia the recommendations are similar but subject to annual review. In cases of acute psychosis or alcohol or opioid dependency a person's licence is revoked for 12 months and they can only resume driving after a drug-free period of 12 months. Regulations for driving a heavy or public vehicle are more stringent, and the counterpart of 12 months in this category is usually 3 years. (Please see www.dvla.gov. uk for more detailed information.)

Chapter 9
Psychiatry and
Neurology

QUESTIONS

THEME: QUESTIONNAIRES

Options

A Audit

B CAGE

C Edinburgh PND scale

D GHQ

E MMSE

F PANSS

G PHQ 9

H PSE

I WAIS

J WAIS-III

For each of the patients below, choose the single most appropriate questionnaire from the list of options above. Each option may be used once, more than once or not at all.

☐ **9.1** A 32-year-old patient attends your surgery and you want to check for alcohol problems.

☐ **9.2** A 32-year-old woman recently gave birth to her first child and you want to screen for postnatal depression.

☐ **9.3** A 78-year-old woman is brought in by her daughter, who feels she is becoming more forgetful.

☐ **9.4** You want to carry out a survey of your local population to screen for general psychiatric morbidity.

☐ **9.5** A 50-year-old man presents with low mood, feeling tired all the time, and difficulty sleeping.

THEME: DEMENTIA AND ORGANIC PSYCHIATRY

Options

A Alzheimer disease

B Binswanger disease

C Delirium

D Frontotemporal dementia

E Huntington disease

F Lewy body dementia

G Parkinson dementia

H Pick disease

I Wilson disease

For each of the patients below, choose the single most appropriate diagnosis from the list of options above. Each option may be used once, more than once or not at all.

☐ **9.6** A 76-year-old patient is recovering from a hip replacement operation in a London hospital. For the past 2 days she has been taking out her fluid line and insisting on going to Ireland. The nurses have noticed that her symptoms are worse in the evening.

☐ **9.7** A 76-year-old man with a history of fluctuating consciousness and visual hallucinations became extremely stiff and had a fall after being given 0.5 mg risperidone to treat his hallucinations.

☐ **9.8** An 80-year-old woman lives alone. She is finding it difficult to remember names. Recently she had to be collected from the police station after she lost her way back from the supermarket.

☐ **9.9** A 59-year old man has been seen behaving inappropriately over the past 2 months and has recently exposed himself in public. Recently, he has also been observed to be incontinent.

☐ **9.10** A 37-year-old man has been seen behaving oddly, with abnormal movements and memory problems. On investigation, his liver function tests were found to be compromised.

THEME: SIDE-EFFECTS OF DRUGS

Options

A   Arrhythmia

B   Bone marrow suppression

C   Cheese reaction

D   Discontinuation syndrome

E   Hypothyroidism

F   Liver dysfunction

G   Neural tube abnormalities

H   Neuroleptic malignant syndrome

I   Neutropenia

J   Obesity

K   Serotonin syndrome

For each of the patients below, choose the single most appropriate side-effect from the list of options above. Each option may be used once, more than once or not at all.

☐ **9.11**   A 34-year-old woman has been taking lithium for the past 4 years.

☐ **9.12**   A 27-year-old woman has developed symptoms of irritability, restlessness, sweating, increased muscle tone and myoclonus while her medications are being switched.

☐ **9.13**   A 29-year-old woman with bipolar affective disorder is taking sodium valproate for prophylaxis of her illness. This poses a risk if she gets pregnant.

☐ **9.14**   A risk one should be aware of in a 62-year-old man on amitriptyline.

☐ **9.15**   A side-effect of monoamine oxidase inhibitors (MAOIs) that should be considered.

THEME: DIAGNOSIS OF MENTAL ILLNESS

Options

A Autism

B Bipolar affective disorder

C Catalepsy

D Childhood schizophrenia

E Delirium

F Delirium tremens

G Narcolepsy

H Psychotic depression

I Schizoid personality

J Schizophrenia

K Wernicke's encephalopathy

For each of the patients below, choose the single most appropriate diagnosis from the list of options above. Each option may be used once, more than once or not at all.

☐ 9.16 A 36-year-old man who believes his gut is rotting has not been eating for this reason. He also hears voices saying that he is dead.

☐ 9.17 A 21-year-old-man recently realised, after weeks of having an uneasy feeling and anxiety, that aliens have set up a special link with him to act as a liaison person for planet earth.

☐ 9.18 A 7-year-old boy has a peculiar attachment to a chair, has continued nocturnal enuresis, a vocabulary of seven words and avoids eye contact.

☐ 9.19 A 56-year-old-man, admitted to hospital 2 days ago after a road traffic accident, has become increasingly fearful and restless, and is complaining of small people walking along the ceiling. He has a raised pulse rate, fluctuating consciousness and labile blood pressure.

THEME: DRUG MANAGEMENT OF PSYCHIATRIC DISEASE

Options

A Amitriptyline

B Atropine

C Carbamazepine

D Chlordiazepoxide

E Chlorpromazine

F Citalopram

G Lithium carbonate

H Lorazepam

For each of the patients below, select the single most appropriate drug that should be administered from the list of options above. Each option may be used once, more than once or not at all.

☐ **9.20** A 63-year-old man presents in an agitated state with confusion and visual hallucinations that terrify him. He has pyrexia, tremor and tachycardia and is sweating profusely. He has previously been admitted repeatedly with symptoms associated with chronic alcoholism.

☐ **9.21** A 30-year-old woman is brought to the surgery in an agitated and distractible state. She is in an expansive euphoric mood and will not stop talking. Her friends report that her agitated and excitable behaviour has recently resulted in dismissal from her job.

☐ **9.22** An 83-year old man gives a 3-month history of increasing insomnia, fatigue and difficulty concentrating. He has lost interest in daily activities and feels a burden on his family.

☐ **9.23** The police bring a 45-year-old man to casualty as he has been threatening staff at a nearby store. He has prominent third-person auditory hallucinations and states that the Queen of England, via a radiotransmitter implanted in his teeth, controls his actions.

THEME: HEADACHE

Options

A   Bacterial meningitis

B   Basilar migraine

C   Benign intracranial hypertension

D   Cerebrovascular accident

E   Chronic subdural haematoma

F   Cryptococcal meningitis

G   Herpes encephalitis

H   Normal-pressure hydrocephalus

I   Subarachnoid haemorrhage

J   Transient ischaemic attack

For each of the clinical scenarios below, which one of the list of options above would be the most appropriate cause of headache? Each option may be used once, more than once or not at all.

☐ **9.24** A 75-year-old woman is brought into the surgery with a history of headache, forgetfulness and urinary incontinence for the preceding three weeks.

☐ **9.25** A 23-year-old man has mild headache, low-grade fever and malaise. He has been unwell for 5 days. On examination you notice facial molluscum contagiosum.

☐ **9.26** A 36-year-old man has sudden-onset of the worst headache he has ever experienced. The pain is mostly occipital and he has a reduced Glasgow Coma Scale score.

☐ **9.27** A 19-year-old female university student has fever, headache and cervical rigidity.

☐ **9.28** A 28-year-old rugby player presents to the surgery midway through the season with a 2-week history of ataxia and difficulty passing urine.

☐ **9.29** An obese 29-year-old woman presents with a 3-month history of recurrent headaches and associated visual disturbance. She takes an oral contraceptive and on examination she is noted to have papilloedema.

9.30 The parents of a 4-year-old boy report that he wakes and, at times, screams in the middle of the night. However, he goes back to sleep on his own and has no recollection of the events the following day. His father is known to have had similar experiences as a child.

What is the single most likely diagnosis from the list below?

- ☐ **A** Childhood depression
- ☐ **B** Ill-informed dreams
- ☐ **C** Nightmares
- ☐ **D** Night terrors
- ☐ **E** Somnambulism

9.31 A 24-year-old mother has brought her 2-year-old son to the hospital with diarrhoea. The staff recognise her from her numerous past visits, which have led to several admissions of the boy and, earlier, his older sister. Both are known to have recovered promptly on admission. She is known to have trained as a nurse.

Which one of the following diagnoses is the most likely?

- ☐ **A** Child abuse
- ☐ **B** Failure to thrive
- ☐ **C** Munchhausen syndrome by proxy
- ☐ **D** Non-accidental injury
- ☐ **E** Physical abuse

9.32 A 24-year-old woman presents with a sudden-onset, severe headache with retro-orbital pain and photophobia, associated with two episodes of vomiting. She says it is the worst headache she has ever had. There is no past history of migraine. Examination reveals no neurological deficit.

What is the single most appropriate initial investigation from list below?

- ☐ **A** Computed tomography (CT) scan of the head
- ☐ **B** Erythrocyte sedimentation rate (ESR)
- ☐ **C** Lumbar puncture
- ☐ **D** Magnetic resonance imaging (MRI) of the head
- ☐ **E** Technetium brain scan

9.33 A 46-year-old woman has persistent morning headaches and vomiting. A CT scan shows a space-occupying lesion in the temporal lobe. Assessment of her visual fields reveals a defect.

What is the single most likely defect from the options below?

- ☐ **A** Bitemporal hemianopia
- ☐ **B** Homonymous hemianopia
- ☐ **C** Homonymous lower quadrantic defect
- ☐ **D** Homonymous upper quadrantic defect
- ☐ **E** Unilateral visual loss

ANSWERS

THEME: QUESTIONNAIRES

9.1   B   CAGE

This is a screening questionnaire devised to identify problematic drinking in an outpatient department or primary care setting. It comprises a four-item questionnaire about: Cutting down drinking; Annoyed by criticism; Guilty about drinking; Eye-opener drink – needing a drink first thing in the morning. Positive answers to two or more questions are indicative of problem drinking.

9.2   C   Edinburgh PND scale

The Edinburgh Post-Natal Depression scale is a 10-item self-reporting questionnaire used to screen for postnatal depression.

9.3   E   MMSE

The Mini-Mental State Examination is a 30-item objective assessment test that can be used to screen for Alzheimer disease (AD) as well as to monitor prognosis. A score below 26 is usually indicative of mild AD. Recent National Institute for Health and Clinical Excellence (NICE) guidelines (www.nice. org.uk/cg42) recommend the prescription of anti-dementia medication for patients with MMSE scores between 20 and 10.

9.4   D   GHQ

The General Health Questionnaire is a screening tool devised to identify psychiatric morbidity in a population.

9.5   G   PHQ 9

All new diagnoses of depression should have an assessment of severity, on which to base management decisions and monitor progress. Several questionnaires have been recommended for this purpose including the Patient Health Questionnaire (PHQ), part 9 of which measures depression symptoms. Another is the Beck Depression Inventory (BDI), a self-reporting questionnaire.

The acronym AUDIT stands for Alcohol-Use Disorder Identification Test, which was devised by the World Health Organization and is more sensitive than CAGE. PSE stands for Present State Examination and GHQ for General Health Questionnaire, and both these instruments are used to identify psychiatric morbidity. PANSS is Positive And Negative Syndrome Scale and is used for identifying positive and negative symptoms of schizophrenia.

The Wechsler Adult Intelligence Scale-III is valid for use with 5–15-year-olds, whereas WAIS is designed for 16–89-year-olds. It is the most commonly used intelligence test, and has a variety of sub-tests that are divided into 'performance' and 'verbal' domains.

THEME: DEMENTIA AND ORGANIC PSYCHIATRY

9.6   C   Delirium

This is also called 'acute confusional state', and is often associated with the phenomenon of 'sundowning' as described in the scenario.

9.7   F   Lewy body dementia

The classic triad of Lewy body dementia consists of fluctuating consciousness, visual hallucinations and spontaneous parkinsonism. Patients are very susceptible to extrapyramidal symptoms on relatively small doses of neuroleptics, which can be serious. Lewy bodies are found extensively in the cortex (in Parkinson's disease more around the substantia nigra in the subcortical region). Although cholinesterase inhibitors have been found to be effective, they are not yet licensed for this use.

9.8   A   Alzheimer disease

Remember the four As of classic dementia: Amnesia, Agnosia, Aphasia and Apraxia.

9.9   D   Frontotemporal dementia

Pick disease is a particular and rare variant of frontotemporal dementia but the latter has a relatively earlier age of onset.

9.10   I   Wilson disease

Always suspect Huntington disease or Wilson disease in dementia of early onset associated with movement disorder; suspect in early-onset dementia as well (not associated with movement disorders). Family history and genetic counselling are of great importance.

NB: Binswanger disease is also called 'progressive small-vessel disease' – a subcortical dementia associated with cognitive slowing.

THEME: SIDE-EFFECTS OF DRUGS

9.11   E   Hypothyroidism

Lithium can cause thyroid disorders and therefore the *British National Formulary* recommends that thyroid function should be measured every 6–12 months. Also note that lithium has a narrow therapeutic index and serum lithium levels should be monitored to maintain them at 0.4–1.0 mmol/l. Levels above 1.5 mmol/l are dangerous and are associated with coarse tremors, ataxia, renal impairment and convulsions. In this situation, lithium should be withdrawn immediately, and sodium-rich fluid administered to reverse its effects. If levels are over 2 mmol/l, then treatment should be carried out in an intensive care setting.

9.12 K Serotonin syndrome

The symptoms described in the scenario are characteristic of the serotonin syndrome, common when two serotonin reuptake inhibitors (SSRIs) are simultaneously administered, eg switching antidepressants. The symptoms overlap with those of neuroleptic malignant syndrome and can, albeit rarely, be fatal. (See the *British National Formulary*.)

9.13 G Neural tube abnormalities

There is an increased risk of neural tube defects in babies born to mothers taking valproate (also occurs with those on carbamazepine or other antiepileptics). Folic acid supplementation is therefore advised before and during pregnancy to counteract this risk.

9.14 A Arrhythmia

Electrocardiogram (ECG) monitoring is recommended as arrhythmias are a major risk with amitriptyline, and are also associated with abrupt withdrawal of the medication. Other side-effects include urinary retention, closed-angle closure glaucoma and postural hypotension. Liver dysfunction should ring a cautionary bell for many medications, including amitriptyline, but is less specific. Liver dysfunction can sometimes occur but hepatic failure is not common.

9.15 C Cheese reaction

MAOIs are inhibitors of monoamine oxidase. They inhibit the metabolism of monoamine-containing drugs (eg decongestants and cough preparations) as well as foods rich in tyramine (mature cheese, pickled herring, broad beans, etc). This causes the accumulation of amines and results in dangerous rise of blood pressure – the 'cheese reaction'. The effects persist for up to 2 weeks after taking an MAOI.

THEME: DIAGNOSIS OF MENTAL ILLNESS

9.16   H   Psychotic depression

The symptoms described are typical of nihilistic delusion. Nihilistic delusions are pessimistic delusions, eg one is going to die, or even a part of the body is dead, one has no money or the world is coming to an end. Nihilistic delusions are associated with extremes of depressed mood, and respond to treatment of the underlying depression although antipsychotics are often required in the short term.

9.17   J   Schizophrenia

This disorder has a heterogeneous presentation. Symptoms can be clustered into those in which there is loss of a sense of reality, and those of disorganisation and apathy (the latter are the negative symptoms). The reality distortions include delusions or faulty beliefs, and hallucinations or faulty perceptions, and together these comprise the positive symptoms (a more specific list is included in the classification of symptoms for diagnosis). The symptom described here is suggestive of what can be considered as bizarre delusion and also hints towards thought-broadcast experience, both of which are included in the diagnostic criteria given in *International Classification of Diseases 10th Revision* (ICD-10) and *Diagnostic and Statistical Manual of Mental Disorders IV* (DSM-IV).

9.18   A   Autism

Autism is a disorder that presents with three clusters of features: difficulties in social relationships, difficulties with language development and ritualistic tendencies. It is often associated with abnormal attachment to inanimate objects and developmental delays. The nocturnal enuresis is suggestive of a generalised developmental delay, as in this case.

9.19 F Delirium tremens

Delirium tremens is precipitated within 48–72 hours of abstinence in a chronic heavy drinker, and is commonly seen after emergency hospital admission where a background history of alcohol use is often unavailable. Vivid hallucinations, particularly visual hallucinations involving lilliputian images, are classic. However, tactile or auditory hallucinations are not uncommon. Fearful affect, perceptual misinterpretations and delusions are common. There is disorientation and fluctuating consciousness with autonomic hyperactivity. Delirium is a blanket diagnosis that would cover delirium tremens, but it is less specific and therefore not the 'most likely' answer.

THEME: DRUG MANAGEMENT OF PSYCHIATRIC DISEASE

9.20 D Chlordiazepoxide

Delirium tremens typically presents acutely after 3–4 days of abstinence from alcohol. When fully developed the syndrome includes vivid visual hallucinations (not definitely required for the diagnosis), delusions, confusion, agitation and autonomic arousal (often including pyrexia). While short lived (a few days), mortality can be up to 20%. Treatment is fluid replacement and sedation with diazepam or chlordiazepoxide with close monitoring for electrolyte imbalance (especially hypokalaemia).

9.21   H   Lorazepam

Bipolar disorders consist of marked changes in mood that vary from major depressive episodes to major manic episodes. A manic episode consists of a sustained period (at least a week) when mood was abnormally and persistently elevated, expansive or irritable. Symptoms include inflated self-esteem (which may be delusional), decreased need for sleep, talkativeness, flight of ideas, distractibility; they typically cause marked impairment in occupational functioning or relationships with others. The average age of onset of bipolar disorder is about 30 years. Treatment of the acute manic phase is often in hospital. Lithium is not useful in the acute phase of mania, with benzodiazepines (especially lorazepam) being used instead. If the agitation is marked and uncontrolled with medication, it is possible to use electroconvulsive treatment to control the manic excitement.

9.22   F   Citalopram

Symptoms of depression are the commonest psychiatric symptoms in community samples of elderly adults. As with all depressive symptoms, when symptoms become more marked, particularly when disturbing sleep or appetite, then antidepressant medications should be used. In patients who present primarily with insomnia (or agitation), amitriptyline is sometimes used for its sedating effects, particularly given at bedtime. However tricyclics are associated with arrhythmias and should be avoided in the elderly or patients with cardiovascular disease. The tricyclics are also more dangerous in overdose, so suicide risk should be frequently assessed. The most likely first choice in this scenario would be citalopram, as it is a serotonin selective reuptake inhibitor (SSRI) with sedative properties. The SSRIs have a much better safety profile in this age group.

CHAPTER 9 ANSWERS

9.23   E   Chlorpromazine

Schizophrenia is characterized by psychotic symptoms during the active phase of the illness. Symptoms include bizarre delusions (eg involving a phenomenon that the individual's culture would regard as totally implausible such as thoughts being broadcast out loud), prominent hallucinations (often a voice commenting on the individual's behaviour or thoughts), incoherent speech, catatonic behaviour and flat or inappropriate affect. During the course of the illness, there is significant deterioration in social functioning and self-care. The goal of treatment initially is to decrease symptom occurrence. Medication dosage is increased as long as hallucinations, delusions and disorganised thinking continue; the most frequent limiting factor is the appearance of extrapyramidal side-effects.

THEME: HEADACHE

9.24   H   Normal-pressure hydrocephalus

This is usually a disorder of the elderly. There is enlargement of the cerebral ventricles without an increase in the cerebrospinal fluid pressure. It commonly presents with dementia, ataxia and urinary incontinence.

9.25   F   Cryptococcal meningitis

This is an acquired immune deficiency syndrome (AIDS)-defining illness. It occurs in patients with a low CD4 count. It often has a slowly evolving prodromal phase with fever, malaise and headache. Patients may have nausea, vomiting and photophobia and neck stiffness at the time of presentation. Indian-ink staining of the cerebrospinal fluid shows *Cryptococcus neoformans*. Treatment is with the intravenous antifungal agents amphotericin and/or flucytosine. Facial molluscum contagiosum is a good indicator of immunosuppression in HIV infection.

9.26   I   Subarachnoid haemorrhage

This patient has had a spontaneous bleed into the subarachnoid space. It classically presents with very severe headache of sudden onset. The initial pain is often in the occipital region. Patients may remain well or be very seriously ill on presentation. Diagnosis is by CT scan or lumbar puncture if the CT scan is negative and no focal lesion is demonstrated. It is often associated with underlying saccular (berry) aneurysms or arteriovenous (AV) malformations.

9.27   A   Bacterial meningitis

This girl has bacterial meningitis. She has the classic signs of fever, headache and neck stiffness. Photophobia and vomiting are often present. Meningococcal (*Neisseria meningitidis*) meningitis should be immediately suspected. There may or may not be a petechial rash. Cefotaxime/ceftriaxone therapy should be commenced as soon as possible if meningococcal meningitis is thought to likely. This disease may show rapid progression from being fully well to septicaemia and the value of early antibiotics should not be underestimated. Lumbar puncture should be avoided.

9.28   E   Chronic subdural haematoma

This is caused by slow bleeding from a vein into the subdural space. Gradually symptoms result from haematoma accumulation over a period of days or weeks. There may be headache, reduced mental capacity or more focal signs. Elderly people and alcohol misusers are at highest risk but trauma can be a cause in any age group.

9.29   C   Benign intracranial hypertension

This uncommon disorder often occurs in overweight women. It represents an increase in cerebrospinal fluid pressure without an increase in the size of the cerebral ventricles. It causes headache and visual blurring due to papilloedema. It may be associated with steroids and tetracycline treatment. Thiazide diuretics and acetazolamide may be useful in management. Weight reduction may also be helpful.

CHAPTER 9 ANSWERS

9.30   D   Night terrors

Somnambulism is sleep-walking and the main concern in its management is safety. Both somnambulism and night terrors are more common in children, occur in non-REM sleep and are known to have a strong familial component. Dreams in the non-REM phase are ill-formed and often not recollected. On the other hand, nightmares occur during REM sleep.

9.31   C   Munchhausen syndrome by proxy

Although this can be classified as non-accidental injury and physical/child misuse, a presentation such as the one described is unique (and rare) and known as 'Munchhausen syndrome by proxy'. This syndrome manifests as repeated presentations by a parent complaining that their child is ill. At times, the illness is induced or fabricated. Adults similarly presenting themselves have 'Munchhausen syndrome', which is considered a factitious illness, with no obvious gain. This is a serious and rare matter, and should be dealt with sensitively with child protection in mind.

9.32   A   CT scan of the head

CT imaging is the initial investigation of choice, which usually shows the presence of subarachnoid or intraventricular blood. A lumbar puncture is unnecessary if a subarachnoid haemorrhage is confirmed by CT, but should be considered if doubt remains. The CSF becomes yellow (xanthochromic) about 12 hours after a subarachnoid haemorrhage. MR angiography is usually performed in all patients who are potentially fit for surgery.

9.33   D   Homonymous upper quadrantic defect

Temporal lobe lesions cause an upper quadrantic defect and parietal lobes a lower one. A lesion to the optic chiasma causes bitemporal hemianopia. Optic tract lesions cause field defects, which are homonymous, hemianopic and often incomplete and incongruous.

Chapter 10
Renal and Urology

QUESTIONS

THEME: LOW URINE OUTPUT AFTER SURGERY

Options

A   Acute interstitial nephritis

B   Acute urinary retention

C   Blocked catheter

D   Chronic kidney disease

E   Renal hypoperfusion due to hypotension

F   Renal hypoperfusion due to intravascular depletion

G   Urinary infection

For each of the following presentations, choose the most likely cause from the list of options above. Each option may be used once, more than once or not at all.

☐ **10.1** An 80-year-old man is usually hypertensive. He is postoperative day 1 following hemicolectomy. He has epidural analgesia for the pain. His urine output reduces after he is given his usual long-term medication.

☐ **10.2** A 65-year-old man has undergone hernia repair as a day case. He has not passed urine since the procedure, and on examination there is a suprapubic mass.

☐ **10.3** A 73-year-old man has undergone a transurethral resection of the prostate (TURP). In spite of irrigation his urine is heavily blood stained and he is passing < 20ml/h of urine.

☐ **10.4** A 35-year-old man has had a subtotal colectomy for ulcerative colitis. He has been given gentamicin as prophylaxis and diclofenac for analgesia. On the first postoperative day his urine output has tailed off to < 10ml/h.

THEME: IMAGING TECHNIQUES FOR RENAL DISEASES

Options

A   Antegrade pyelography
B   Computed tomography (CT) scan
C   Dipstick urinalysis
D   Micturating cystography
E   Magnetic resonance imaging (MRI)
F   Plain X-ray
G   Renal arteriography
H   Renal biopsy
I   Renal scintigraphy
J   Retrograde pyelography
K   Ultrasound scan

For each of the case scenarios below, choose the most appropriate investigation from the list of options above. Each option may be used once, more than once or not at all.

☐ **10.5** This investigation would be needed to diagnose the problem in a patient who had rising urea and creatinine levels after taking an angiotensin-converting enzyme (ACE) inhibitor for a couple of weeks.

☐ **10.6** This is a useful investigation for recurrent urinary tract infection, especially in adults with disturbed bladder function. It can be combined with urodynamic measurements of bladder pressure and urethral flow.

☐ **10.7** A useful investigation for patients with suspected ureteric colic who have no stones visible on ultrasound or plain abdominal X-ray.

☐ **10.8** This is the investigation of choice for diagnosing polycystic kidney disease, measuring renal size and detecting renal vein thrombosis.

THEME: DIAGNOSIS OF RENAL DISEASE

Options

A Acute tubulointerstitial nephritis

B Analgesic nephropathy

C Contrast medium induced nephropathy

D Haemolytic uraemic syndrome

E Idiopathic thrombocytopenic purpura

F IgA nephropathy

G Medullary cystic kidney disease

H Retroperitoneal fibrosis

I Streptococcal glomerulonephritis

For each of the patients below, choose the most likely diagnosis from the list of options above. Each option may be used once, more than once or not at all.

☐ **10.9** A 10-year-old boy has had a sore throat, which he thinks he caught from his friend who returned from Africa last week. His parents think his limbs are starting to swell, and this morning he told them his urine was red. On bedside urine testing there is blood and protein in his urine.

☐ **10.10** A 48-year-old woman has noticed recent ankle swelling, a feeling of abdominal bloating, and she thinks she is passing less urine than usual. She recently had a CT scan.

☐ **10.11** A 5-year-old girl experiences an episode of severe diarrhoea following a recent school trip to a farm. She now has haematuria and her blood results show thrombocytopenia and her urea and electrolytes are rising.

☐ **10.12** A 62-year-old man with a previous history of surgery for abdominal aortic aneurysm presented with malaise, backache and normochromic anaemia, uraemia and a raised erythrocyte sedimentation rate (ESR). A peri-aortic mass is seen on CT.

THEME: MANAGEMENT OF ACUTE RENAL FAILURE

Options

A Angiotensin-converting enzyme (ACE) inhibitor

B Calcium resonium orally/per rectum

C Catheterisation

D Continuous ambulatory peritoneal dialysis (CAPD)

E Haemodilution

F Haemofiltration

G Intravenous calcium gluconate

H Insulin plus dextrose

I Intravenous fluid

J Intravenous furosemide

For each of the patients below, choose the most appropriate management option from the list above. Each option may be used once, more than once or not at all.

☐ **10.13** A 64-year-old man with end-stage renal disease, limited exercise tolerance due to chronic obstructive pulmonary disease and a colostomy due to a past history of ulcerative colitis has acute deterioration in his renal function.

☐ **10.14** An 85-year-old man presents with anuria for the past 72 hours. He is confused and restless. Examination reveals a distended lower abdomen and bi-basal chest crepitations. His potassium is 5.8 mmol/l, urea 40 mmol/l and creatinine 760 µmol/l.

10.15 A 42-year-old previously fit and healthy man presents with a traumatic fractured neck of femur. A large haematoma is drained during surgery. Since the operation he has had episodes of vomiting and complains of thirst and malaise. His blood tests reveal sodium 152 mmol/l, potassium 3.4 mmol/l, urea 26 mmol/l and creatinine 176 μmol/l. (normal values: sodium 135–145 mmol/l, potassium 3.5–5.0 mmol/l, urea 2.5–6.7 mmol/l and creatinine 70–< 150 μmol/l).

10.16 A 62-year-old man with severe cardiovascular disease is taking perindopril, furosemide, spironolactone and carvedilol for heart failure. His potassium level has been slowly rising and has been 6.5 mmol/l for the past few weeks. The cardiologists are reluctant to change his heart failure medications as this regimen seems to have optimised his cardiac function. However they wish to deal with his potassium level before it goes any higher. He is asymptomatic with no changes on electrocardiography.

THEME: MANAGEMENT OF CHRONIC KIDNEY DISEASE

Options

A   Angiotensin-converting enzyme (ACE) inhibitor

B   β-Blocker

C   Calcium/cholecalciferol supplements

D   Erythropoiesis stimulating agents

E   Giovannetti diet

F   Granulocyte colony stimulating factor

G   Oral phosphodiesterase inhibitor

H   Pneumococcal vaccine

For each of the patients below, choose the most appropriate management option from the list of options above. Each option may be used once, more than once or not at all.

☐ **10.17** A 60-year-old man is diagnosed as having stage 3 chronic kidney disease (CKD). His parathormone (PTH) level is raised and 25-hydroxyvitamin D level is low.

☐ **10.18** A 72-year-old man has routine monitoring of haemoglobin, potassium, calcium and phosphate for stage 3 CKD. His haemoglobin is found to be 9.0 g/l (normal 13.5–18 g/l). Investigations for occult bleeding are negative. He is getting too breathless to walk upstairs, and has started sleeping downstairs.

☐ **10.19** A 78-year-old woman has just been diagnosed with stage 3 CKD. Her medications include alendronate, Calcichew D3 (calcium salt), lisinopril and omeprazole. She does not have any symptoms at present.

☐ **10.20** A 65-year-old man receiving continuous ambulatory peritoneal dialysis (CAPD) for hypertensive nephropathy complains of distressing impotence. There is no history of coronary artery disease.

THEME: INCONTINENCE

Options

A Anticholinergics

B Bladder training

C Catheter

D Colposuspension operation

E Cystoscopy

F Frequency/volume chart

G Midstream sample of urine

H Pad collection of urine

I Pelvic floor exercises

For each clinical scenario below, choose the most appropriate next step in management from the list of options above. Each option may be used once, more than once or not at all.

☐ **10.21** A 23-year-old woman presents with a 3-day history of frequency and dysuria. A couple of times she waited too long to pass urine and found she did not quite make it to the toilet before suddenly losing control.

☐ **10.22** A 38-year-old woman had her third baby by vaginal delivery 6 months ago. She complains of leaking small amounts of urine whenever she coughs or sneezes.

☐ **10.23** An 80-year-old man has been complaining of longstanding constipation. After many months of laxatives this seems to be improving, but during this time he has developed urinary incontinence. He tells you he passes urine every half an hour during the day, and is getting up several times in the night. He is being treated for benign prostatic hypertrophy and now has a good urinary flow.

☐ **10.24** A 75-year-old woman complains of needing to wear a pad day and night due to urinary incontinence. It happens without warning but more so if she strains or bends down. She has tried pelvic floor exercises for more than 3 months, and is intolerant of medication.

THEME: PRESCRIBING FOR PATIENTS IN RENAL FAILURE

Options

A   Absolutely contraindicated

B   Higher doses may be needed

C   Monitor drug levels more often

D   No changes required

E   Reduce dose

F   Reduced dose frequency

G   Relatively contraindicated

For each drug below, choose the most appropriate advice from the list of options above. Each option may be used once, more than once or not at all.

☐ **10.25** Captopril in moderate renal impairment

☐ **10.26** Gentamicin in severe chronic renal impairment

☐ **10.27** Furosemide for pulmonary oedema in severe acute renal failure

☐ **10.28** Phenytoin in severe renal impairment

☐ **10.29** Cefalexin in severe chronic renal impairment

10.30 A 56-year-old man has been treated for many years with felodipine for hypertension. Now this is not adequately controlling his blood pressure and angiotensin-converting enzyme (ACE) inhibitor treatment is planned. On routine baseline blood tests prior to commencing treatment the estimated glomerular filtration rate (eGFR) is 49 ml/min/1.73m^2 (normal > 90 ml/min/1.73m^2).

From the following list of options choose the single most appropriate next step in his management.

- [ ] **A** Commence the ACE inhibitor as planned
- [ ] **B** Examine the patient, and do urinalysis
- [ ] **C** Recheck blood tests in 2 weeks
- [ ] **D** Refer him to the on-call medic for immediate admission
- [ ] **E** Refer to the local nephrology outpatients

10.31 A 4-year-old boy complains that the end of his penis 'balloons' when he passes urine. His parents tell you the flow of urine is quite poor when this happens, and that it is happening more often as time goes by. They ask if he needs circumcision. On gentle examination his foreskin is easily retracted and replaced.

From the following list of options, choose the single most likely diagnosis.

- [ ] **A** Balanitis
- [ ] **B** Non-retractile foreskin
- [ ] **C** Paraphimosis
- [ ] **D** Peyronie disease
- [ ] **E** Phimosis

10.32 A 36-year-old man presents with a painless lump in his scrotum. He is otherwise well, but his mother had ovarian cancer and he is very concerned. On supine examination the scrotum is not inflamed, both testes are of normal size and shape, non-tender, and there is a pea-sized lump behind his left testis. It feels integral to the rope-like structure running along the back of each testis. There is no inguinal lymphadenopathy.

From the following list of options, choose the single most likely diagnosis.

- [ ] **A** Epididymal cyst
- [ ] **B** Epididymo-orchitis
- [ ] **C** Hydrocele
- [ ] **D** Testicular cancer
- [ ] **E** Varicocele

ANSWERS

THEME: LOW URINE OUTPUT AFTER SURGERY

10.1   E   Renal hypoperfusion due to hypotension

Epidural analgesia can reduce the blood pressure. This patient's usual dose of antihypertensive medication reduced the blood pressure even further, in this case leading to hypoperfusion of the kidneys which then produce less urine.

10.2   B   Acute urinary retention

Some older men will develop acute urinary retention following routine inguinal hernia surgery. This is thought to be due to a combination of prostatic hypertrophy and the anticholinergic effects of some anaesthetic reversal agents. Pain may also contribute. A brief period of catheterisation will usually be sufficient to treat the acute episode.

10.3   C   Blocked catheter

Clot retention is a common problem following TURP and often responds to bladder washout under strict aseptic technique. Rarely patients may need to return to theatre for further haemostatic diathermy.

10.4   A   Acute interstitial nephritis

Aminoglycoside antibiotics such as gentamicin can be nephrotoxic, as can non-steroidal anti-inflammatory drugs such as diclofenac. They can lead to acute renal failure due to interstitial nephritis. Risk factors for these effects include dehydration, hypotension, pre-existing renal impairment and the concomitant use of multiple nephrotoxic drugs.

THEME: IMAGING TECHNIQUES FOR RENAL DISEASES

10.5   G   Renal arteriography

When starting to take ACE inhibitors, patients should be advised that they will need to have blood tests for urea and creatinine at baseline, which will need to be repeated a week or two after starting the drug or following any dose increase. This is to monitor for the rare condition of renal artery stenosis, which can be revealed by ACE inhibitors (or angiotensin II receptor blockers). Patients with deteriorating urea and electrolyte findings should be investigated with renal arteriography to detect underlying arterial stenosis, as this can lead to chronic kidney disease if left undetected.

10.6   D   Micturating cystography

The patient is screened during voiding after a contrast agent has been instilled into the bladder. This is to check for vesicoureteric reflux and to study urethral and bladder emptying.

10.7   B   CT scan

CT can be used to detect lucent calculi. It is also used as first line to characterise renal masses that are indeterminate on ultrasound screening, for staging of renal tumours, evaluation of the retroperitoneum for tumours or fibrosis (that may be causing renal obstruction), assessment of renal trauma, and visualisation of renal vasculature.

10.8   K   Ultrasound scan

Ultrasound is also useful for checking whether renal masses are solid or cystic, detecting infrarenal or perinephric fluid, and for demonstrating renal perfusion.

THEME: DIAGNOSIS OF RENAL DISEASE

10.9   I   Streptococcal glomerulonephritis

The incidence of streptococcal glomerulonephritis is declining in the West, but it is still prevalent in some parts of the world, particularly in tropical countries. This is because it is due to the deposition of immune complexes in the glomeruli following infection with certain serotypes of *Streptococcus* that are mainly seen in those areas. It is not known why some people infected with the same serotypes do not have any sequelae. The condition typically affects children between 2 and 12 years.

10.10   C   Contrast medium induced nephropathy

Some people are sensitive to the agents used as radiographic contrast. If someone has had recent investigations it is worth checking if they were given any injections during the procedure. Reactions can worsen on subsequent exposure, so patients should be clearly told to let radiographers know about this if they should need investigations in the future.

10.11   D   Haemolytic uraemic syndrome

Certain pathogens, including *Escherichia coli* serotype O157, can produce 'verotoxins' that damage endothelial cells. This leads to platelet and fibrin deposition in small vessels, causing intravascular haemolysis. This is also known as microangiopathic haemolytic anaemia. The platelets are used up in the process (consumptive thrombocytopenia), and red cell degradation products damage the kidneys. It is a disease primarily of infancy and early childhood, and is the most common cause of acute renal failure in children.

10.12   H   Retroperitoneal fibrosis

This condition may extend from the level of the second lumbar vertebra to the pelvic brim. It is thought to be due to an autoimmune phenomenon. There is an association sometimes with abdominal aortic aneurysm but most cases are idiopathic. The differential diagnosis is retroperitoneal lymphoma.

THEME: MANAGEMENT OF ACUTE RENAL FAILURE

10.13   F   Haemofiltration

This patient can no longer be managed conservatively and needs to have more invasive treatment. His previous surgery makes CAPD unsuitable for him therefore haemodialysis is the modality of choice.

10.14   C   Catheterisation

The patient's symptoms and biochemistry results are consistent with acute urinary retention causing obstructive uropathy. This may have been precipitated by treatment with diuretics for his heart failure, or a urinary tract infection. A brief period of catheterisation and careful fluid balance will usually help the renal function slowly return to his normal status.

10.15   I   Intravenous fluid

A large volume of fluid loss without adequate replacement can result in 'prerenal' acute renal failure. This can be corrected by judicious fluid replacement.

10.16   B   Calcium resonium orally/per rectum

An ion-exchange resin such as calcium resonium can lower the potassium if the medications causing high levels cannot be stopped. If the patient had symptoms or there were electrocardiographic effects of hyperkalaemia he would need admission for intravenous treatment. However with adequate monitoring, the oral or rectal route is acceptable in this situation.

THEME: MANAGEMENT OF CHRONIC KIDNEY DISEASE

10.17   C   Calcium/cholecalciferol supplements

At first diagnosis of stage 3 CKD, the PTH should be checked, and if it is raised the 25-hydroxyvitamin D should be checked. If this is low the patient should be started on ergo- or cholecalciferol plus calcium supplements (not calcium phosphate) in an attempt to maintain serum calcium concentrations in the normal range and prevent excess parathormone secretion.

10.18   D   Erythropoiesis stimulating agents

The renal production of erythropoietin is reduced in CKD, therefore patients should be monitored for anaemia. In the absence of any other cause they should be treated with erythropoiesis stimulating agents (eg epoetin or darbepoetin alfa) to maintain the haemoglobin between 11.0 g/l and 12.0 g/l, depending on functional needs. These agents have side-effects such as causing hypertension, and patients need to be monitored for this and treated accordingly.

10.19   H   Pneumococcal vaccine

Once a patient is diagnosed with CKD stage 3 or above they should have their medications and vaccinations reviewed. Nephrotoxic drugs including non-steroidal anti-inflammatory drugs should be avoided if possible, and if they have never had a pneumococcal vaccine this should be given as a single dose. They should also receive annual influenza vaccination.

10.20   G   Oral phosphodiesterase inhibitor

Phosphodiesterase inhibitors such as sildenafil can be effective in treating erectile dysfunction in patients with renal failure. These drugs are contraindicated in those receiving treatment with nitrates for coronary artery disease.

THEME: INCONTINENCE

10.21   G   Midstream sample of urine

Frequency and dysuria are classic symptoms of urinary tract infection. Occasionally the infection can cause detrusor irritability leading to urge incontinence. Treatment involves eradicating the infection. Unless the patient tells you she frequently suffers from cystitis it is appropriate to send a midstream sample of urine for culture and sensitivities prior to commencing empirical treatment.

10.22   I   Pelvic floor exercises

Following vaginal delivery, particularly if instrumental, there is damage to the pelvic floor muscles, which become overstretched and lax. It is important to advise the woman *how* to perform pelvic floor exercises, including giving information sheets with instructions.

10.23   B   Bladder training

Faecal overloading due to constipation can cause bladder outflow obstruction, leading to incomplete bladder emptying, frequency of micturition and sometimes overflow incontinence. Even though the obstruction has now cleared the bladder may take some time to get used to holding urine for longer periods once more. Bladder training, to extend the time between voids, can help this problem.

10.24   D   Colposuspension operation

In this situation it is appropriate to try pelvic floor exercises first, and then medication if this is unsuccessful. (See the National Institute for Health and Clinical Excellence (NICE) guidance for the management of urinary incontinence in women (www.nice.org.uk/cg40). A colposuspension procedure can provide support to the bladder neck and treat stress incontinence once other options have been exhausted.

THEME: PRESCRIBING FOR PATIENTS IN RENAL FAILURE

The kidneys eliminate many drugs or their metabolites. If renal clearance is reduced, the drug or metabolite may be retained and reach toxic levels. Different drugs are affected in different ways. Less commonly, reduced renal function means a higher dose of a drug is required for it to be effective. This particularly applies to drugs that act on the nephron.

10.25 E Reduce dose

Captopril may become toxic if creatinine clearance is low. The risk of cardiovascular side-effects is greater. The starting dose should be reduced and the patient's renal function should be monitored more regularly. Angiotensin-converting enzyme (ACE) inhibitors are contraindicated in patients with bilateral renal artery stenosis or unilateral renal artery stenosis supplying a single functioning kidney. In these situations, reduction in angiotensin II may lead to rapid deterioration in renal function. Particular care should be taken in prescribing NSAIDs in combination with ACE inhibitors. Creatinine clearance in patients with renal artery stenosis may be well preserved and serum creatinine may be normal. ACE inhibitors are being used increasingly by renal specialists for controlling hypertension in patients with renal disease with good evidence of a protective effect.

10.26 C Monitor drug levels more often

Gentamicin excretion is very sensitive to reduction in renal function. It is also nephrotoxic, especially when given in combination with loop diuretics. Patients should have gentamicin levels monitored routinely. In renal impairment, monitoring should be more frequent and the dose will probably be lower. The loading dose remains the same but the dose and/or the frequency may need adjusting. It is standard practice to measure peak (post-dose) and trough (pre-dose) levels. If the peak levels are high, the dose needs reducing. If the trough levels are high, the frequency needs reducing.

10.27 B Higher dose may be needed

Furosemide acts on the loop of Henle in the nephron. Consequently, if the number of functioning nephrons are reduced, the dose of furosemide may need increasing to achieve the same diuretic effect. It is not uncommon for patients in acute renal failure to be given 250 mg of furosemide over 1 hour in an attempt to start diuresis. It is important to monitor renal function as it may deteriorate with the administration of any diuretic. Higher doses must be given slowly to reduce the risk of drug-induced deafness.

10.28   D   No changes required

Phenytoin is metabolised by the liver and is largely protein bound in the blood. It is unaffected by renal function but may be affected by liver disease or by co-administration of drugs that are also protein bound. Theoretically, in nephrotic syndrome, hypoproteinaemia may affect phenytoin levels.

10.29   F   Reduced dose frequency

Most cephalosporins are excreted unchanged by the kidney and will accumulate in renal failure. Even in mild renal failure, some dose adjustment is required. In most cases, this means a reduction in dose frequency (twice daily instead of three times daily in mild or moderate renal impairment, once daily in severe renal impairment). It is often forgotten that renal function in older patients may be impaired even in the presence of relatively normal creatinine. A 75-year-old of normal body weight with a creatinine of 100 mmol/l will have at least mildly impaired creatinine clearance.

10.30   B   Examine the patient, and do urinalysis

In April 2006 most laboratories started to routinely provide eGFR results with results of urea and electrolyte tests. It forms the basis of our diagnosis of chronic kidney disease (see the National Service Framework for referral criteria). The normal eGFR for a healthy young adult is above 90 ml/min/ 1.73m². However, glomerular filtration rate slows with age, therefore a stable level between 60 ml/min/1.73m² and 90 ml/min/1.73m², with no other signs of kidney disease, may be acceptable and needs no further monitoring. It is calculated from the patient's creatinine. This means it is artificially lower in dehydration (such as during a fasting blood test, therefore advise patients to drink plenty of water).

For this patient it is important to exclude signs of chronic kidney disease such as proteinuria, oedema, enlarged kidneys on palpation, and potential causes of kidney damage such as severe hypertension or outflow obstruction from an enlarged prostate. In the absence of other signs or symptoms it would be appropriate to recheck the blood test in a month to ensure it is stable. This result may indicate his usual level of renal function secondary to long-term hypertension. ACE inhibitors would therefore be appropriate for him to prevent further damage, but should only be started once his baseline renal function is established, as this need to be monitored for any treatment-related deterioration.[3]

10.31   E   Phimosis

In phimosis the foreskin obstructs the flow of urine. It is common in small children and will usually settle with time. Boys should be advised to gently retract the foreskin when passing urine, and ensure that the area is kept clean and dry to avoid balanitis (inflammation of the glans and foreskin). If it persists, or the foreskin becomes non-retractile, or if it causes problems such as recurrent balanitis, the child should be referred to paediatric surgery outpatients.

Paraphimosis is where the foreskin is retracted and becomes oedematous, making it unable to be replaced. It is an emergency and if gentle attempts to replace the foreskin with ice packs (to reduce swelling) and lubricant jelly are unsuccessful the child will require urgent referral.

10.32   A   Epididymal cyst

Epididymal cysts are common and often multiple. They usually present in middle age with a lump as in this case. Management involves reassuring the patient, but they may need an ultrasound if the diagnosis is uncertain. Varicocele causes a dull ache in the testis and is usually only visible when standing.

---

[3] Department of Health. National Service Framework for renal services: Part 2 – chronic kidney disease, Acute renal failure and end of life care. 2005.

Chapter 11
Reproductive

QUESTIONS

THEME: GYNAECOLOGICAL INVESTIGATIONS

Options

A   Cervical punch biopsy

B   Colposcopy and large loop excision of the transformation zone

C   Diagnostic hysteroscopy and endometrial biopsy

D   Diagnostic laparoscopy and tubal dye test

E   Diagnostic laparotomy

F   Hysterosalpingo contrast sonography (HyCoSy)

G   Hysterosalpingography

H   Pregnancy test and serum β-human chorionic gonadotrophin

I   Serum luteinising hormone (LH) and serum follicle-stimulating hormone (FSH)

J   Transabdominal ultrasound of the pelvis

K   Transvaginal ultrasound of the pelvis, Pipelle biopsy and saline sonography

For each of the patients below, choose the single most appropriate investigation from the list of options above. Each option may be used once, more than once or not at all.

☐   **11.1   A 55-year-old woman comes to your clinic with a history of intermenstrual bleeding while on cyclical combined hormone replacement therapy.**

☐ **11.2** A 23-year-old woman is rushed into accident and emergency in a state of shock. Her partner informs you that she had been complaining of lower abdominal pain this morning and then suddenly collapsed. He also tells you that her last menstrual period was 6–7 weeks ago. A portable transabdominal scan (TAS) shows free fluid in the pelvis. On examination her Glasgow Coma Score is 3, pulse is 140 bpm, blood pressure is 70/40 mmHg.

☐ **11.3** A 35-year-old woman comes to your clinic with a 2-year history of primary subfertility. She also gives a history of menstrual irregularity, severe dysmenorrhoea and dyspareunia.

☐ **11.4** A 42-year-old woman comes to your clinic with a 4-year history of secondary infertility. She already has a 6-year-old girl who was conceived through in vitro fertilisation. It has only been recently that she has had the financial means to consider a second child. She also informs you that for the past few months her periods have gradually become more and more irregular and she has also been experiencing night sweats.

☐ **11.5** A 48-year-old asylum seeker presents to your clinic with a history of bloodstained, foul-smelling vaginal discharge. On per speculum examination you see a large ulcerated mass arising from the cervix.

THEME: CONTRACEPTION

Options

A Combined oral contraceptive

B Condoms

C Dianette

D Diaphragm with spermicidal gel

E Implanon

F Injection of Depo-Provera

G Intrauterine copper device

H Lactational amenorrhoea method (LAM)

I Levonorgestrel (morning-after pill)

J Mirena coil

K Progesterone-only pill

For each of the patients below, choose the single most appropriate method of contraception from the list of options above. Each option may be used once, more than once or not at all.

☐ **11.6** A 16-year-old girl comes to your family planning clinic requesting contraceptive advice. She has been sexually active for the past year and is in a stable relationship with her boyfriend. She also informs you that she does not want anything that will make her acne worse.

☐ **11.7** A 26-year-old woman, 7 weeks' postpartum, comes to your family planning clinic for contraceptive advice. While taking a history you gather she is partially breastfeeding, although the vast majority of the feeds are breast feeds. She is not keen on any hormonal contraceptive, as her best friends have told her that they can reduce breast milk.

☐ **11.8** A 24-year-old woman tourist is brought into accident and emergency by the police surgeon who provides information that she was raped 4 days ago. You are asked to perform a medical examination on the patient and advise her about the most suitable contraception. Her last menstrual period was 12 days ago and she has a regular 28-day cycle.

☐ **11.9** A 45-year-old woman is requesting sterilisation. Her history reveals that she has been happily married for the past 20 years and her husband is not keen on a vasectomy. She also tells you that she has recently noticed that her periods have become heavier and puts this down to her increased weight. Her present body mass index (BMI) is 38 kg/m².

☐ **11.10** A 35-year-old woman comes to the family planning clinic requesting contraceptive advice. She has five children and does not want any more. Her last two pregnancies were conceived after contraception failure, while on the pill and the injection. Her records reveal she had tested positive for *Chlamydia* and was seen in the genitourinary medicine clinic 2 years ago.

THEME: INFERTILITY/ASSISTED REPRODUCTIVE TECHNOLOGY

Options

A   Donor insemination

B   Gamete/zygote intrafallopian transfer (GIFT/ZIFT)

C   Intrauterine insemination (IUI)

D   In vitro fertilisation (IVF)

E   IVF with donor egg

F   IVF with intracytoplasmic sperm injection (ICSI)

G   Laparoscopic multi-electrocauterisation of the ovary

H   Ovulation induction with follicular tracking

I   Surrogacy

J   Tubal surgery

For each of the infertile couples below, choose the most appropriate management from the list given above. Each option may be used once, more than once or not at all.

☐ **11.11**   A 38-year-old woman and a 40-year-old man have been married for the past 6 years and have been trying for a baby for the past 3 years. Initial investigations show a normal HyCoSy and endocrine profile for the woman, while the man's semen analysis shows him to have oligoasthenospermia (reduced motility and numbers of sperms).

☐ **11.12**   A 23-year-old woman and a 28-year-old man have a 1-year history of primary infertility. History reveals that the man was diagnosed to have hypospadias as a child.

☐ **11.13**   A 28-year-old woman and a 30-year-old man have an 18-month history of primary infertility. Initial endocrine tests show the woman has anovulatory cycles and her partner's semen analysis is normal.

☐ **11.14** A 30-year-old woman and a 35-year-old man come to your infertility clinic for advice. The woman has lost both fallopian tubes due to ectopic pregnancies.

☐ **11.15** A 30-year-old woman and her 42-year-old partner have a 4-year-old son, and during his birth the woman had a massive haemorrhage due to the placenta praevia and ended up with a caesarean hysterectomy. They now want a second child.

THEME: SEXUALLY TRANSMITTED INFECTIONS

Options

A Chancroid

B Condyloma acuminata

C Gonorrhoea

D Granuloma inguinale

E Hepatitis B

F Hepatitis C

G Herpes simplex

H Herpes zoster

I HIV

J Lymphogranuloma venereum

K Syphilitic primary chancre

For each of the patients below, choose the single most appropriate diagnosis from the list given above. Each option may be used once, more than once or not at all.

☐ **11.16** A 38-year-old asylum seeker from sub-Saharan Africa comes to the genitourinary medicine clinic with a history of a painful ulcer on the prepuce of his penis that he has noticed for the past few days. On examination there is a deep, large ulcer with well-defined margins on the prepuce. There are also a few smaller satellite ulcers on the plans penis with tender swollen inguinal lymph nodes.

☐ **11.17** A 22-year-old truck driver comes to the genitourinary medicine clinic complaining of a flu-like illness with fever, headache and backache. He has noticed a few small, fluid-filled, vesicles on his genital area. He also complains of severe burning during micturition.

☐ **11.18** A 36-year-old homosexual man comes to the genitourinary medicine clinic requesting treatment for the white plaques in his mouth. On examination there are a few bluish-brown nodules on his arm.

☐ **11.19** A 22-year-old woman comes to accident and emergency feeling unwell and with high fever. She give a history of vaginal discharge, dysuria and painful intercourse. On examination there is a large lump in the vulval area, which her GP has diagnosed to be a Bartholin abscess.

☐ **11.20** A 38-year-old intravenous drug user is brought to accident and emergency in a comatose state. On examination there are signs suggestive of chronic liver disease with jaundice and ascites. The results of the tests for viral markers show he is positive for HBsAg and anti-HBe.

THEME: VAGINAL DISCHARGE

Options

A   Atrophic vaginitis

B   Bacterial vaginosis

C   Candidiasis

D   Cervical cancer

E   Ectropion

F   Foreign body

G   Gonorrhoea

H   Mittelschmerz

I   Non-gonococcal urethritis (NGU)

J   *Trichomonas vaginalis* infection

K   Vulvovaginitis

For each of the patients below, choose the single most appropriate diagnosis from the list of options above. Each option may be used once, more than once or not at all.

☐ **11.21 A 5-year-old girl is brought by her mother to the walk-in clinic. The mother informs you that she has been recently noticing a discharge on the girl's undergarments. On examination of the external genitalia you notice it to be red and inflamed.**

☐ **11.22 A 65-year-old woman comes to your gynaecology outpatient clinic to have her ring pessary changed. Her history reveals that although she has been well with regard to her prolapse, she has recently been having some bloodstained discharge.**

☐ **11.23** A 23-year-old woman attends the GP surgery complaining of an itchy vaginal discharge. She is in a stable relationship and does not take any contraceptive pill. On examination you notice red and oedematous labia with white spongy areas.

☐ **11.24** An 18-year-old woman comes to the GP surgery complaining of excessive clear vaginal discharge. She is on the combined pill and describes her symptoms as 'feeling wet all the time'.

☐ **11.25** A 26-year-old woman comes to the clinic complaining of dysuria and painful intercourse. She also says she has been recently getting a funny vaginal discharge. She described it as being frothy with a musty smell, causing intense itching and soreness in her vagina.

THEME: VULVAL DISORDERS

Options

A Behçet's disease

B Candidiasis

C Carcinoma of the vulva

D Condyloma lata

E Herpes simplex

F Leucoplakia

G Lichen sclerosis

H Sebaceous cyst

I Tinea cruris

J Varicose veins

K Vulval abscess

L Vulval psoriasis

M Vulval wart

For each of the patients below, choose the single most appropriate diagnosis from the list of options above. Each option may be used once, more than once or not at all.

☐ **11.26** A 55-year-old woman comes to the outpatient department complaining of vaginal bleeding. She has recently noticed a small ulcer on her genitals. On examination there is an ulcer on the vulva, which has an indurated base and everted margins. Palpation reveals inguinal lymphadenopathy.

☐ **11.27** A 30-year-old 7-month pregnant woman comes to the antenatal clinic complaining of a bluish lump that she has noticed in her vulva. The lump has gradually increased in size but has remained painless.

☐ **11.28** A 28-year-old woman comes to the gynaecology clinic having noticed white patches, which are itchy, on her vulva. On examination you notice the vulval skin to be thickened in the areas with the white patches.

☐ **11.29** A 20-year-old patient, who is 6 months' pregnant, attends the genitourinary medicine clinic having been referred by the community midwife after noticing warty lesions on her vulva. On taking a history you gather she is in a stable relationship and has noticed this growth only in the past few weeks. She has no history of having a sexually transmitted infection in the past.

☐ **11.30** A 32-year-old woman is referred by her GP with a painful vulval swelling, which has become progressively larger and has now burst. On examining her you notice a lump in the labia majora. The lump has a punctum and is discharging foul-smelling pus.

☐ **11.31** A 40-year old woman has well demarcated non-scaly erythema involving the vulva and extending to the intertriginous skin of the groin. She also has thick scaling on the scalp.

THEME: BREAST DISORDERS

Options

A   Acute mastitis

B   Benign breast cyst

C   Breast abscess

D   Breast cancer

E   Duct ectasia

F   Fat necrosis

G   Fibroadenoma

H   Fibroadenosis

I   Galactocele

J   Lipoma

K   Sebaceous cyst

For each of the patients below, choose the single most appropriate diagnosis from the list of options above. Each option may be used once, more than once or not at all.

☐ **11.32** A 28-year-old woman comes to the GP surgery complaining of a lump in her breast. On examination there is a non-tender, firm, mobile mass in the upper right quadrant of her breast.

☐ **11.33** A 65-year-old woman comes to the GP surgery complaining that she recently noticed a change in the shape of her left breast. On examination you notice skin dimpling and a peau d'orange appearance of her skin over the left lower quadrant.

☐ **11.34** A 55-year-old woman comes to her GP surgery complaining that she has recently noticed a change in the shape of her nipple. On examination you note her nipple to be slit-like with no discharge or change in colour.

11.35 A 26-year-old woman comes to accident and emergency complaining of pain in her right breast. On examination you notice severe tenderness and swelling in the peri-areolar area. Her axillary lymph nodes are swollen. Her vital signs are stable, although she is running a high temperature.

11.36 A 33-year-old woman comes to see her GP, worried about lumps in her breast. She is very anxious and informs her GP that recently she has noticed two lumps in her breast. On examination you notice two smooth, well-defined, soft lumps in the outer quadrant of her breast.

11.37 A 26-year-old woman, who is 28 weeks' pregnant, complains of breathlessness during a routine antenatal check-up. On clinical examination everything is normal except she is slightly hyperventilating.

Which one of the following findings would you be surprised to encounter during a normal pregnancy?

- ☐ **A** Decrease in the serum ferritin level
- ☐ **B** Increase in cardiac output
- ☐ **C** Increase in glomerular filtration rate (GFR)
- ☐ **D** Increase in the levels of clotting factors VII, VIII and IX
- ☐ **E** Increase in total lung capacity

11.38 A 26-year-old woman and her 28-year-old partner come to see the GP surgery complaining of primary infertility for 2 years. She gives a history of irregular menstrual cycles.

What one of the following is the single best test to see whether she is ovulating or not?

- ☐ **A** Basal body temperature estimation
- ☐ **B** Cervical fern test
- ☐ **C** Day-2 LH and FSH
- ☐ **D** Day-21 progesterone level
- ☐ **E** Endometrial biopsy

11.39   A 32-year-old pregnant woman presented to her GP with pruritus during the third trimester. Liver biochemistry shows cholestasis.

Which one of the following is the single most likely outcome?

- [ ] **A**   The condition will not resolve after delivery
- [ ] **B**   The fetus will probably be harmed
- [ ] **C**   The ingestion of oestrogen-containing oral contraceptive pills will decrease the risk
- [ ] **D**   The prognosis for the mother is poor
- [ ] **E**   There is a minimal risk of recurrence in subsequent pregnancies

11.40   A 32-year-old woman has a 4-month history of amenorrhoea after stopping the combined oral contraceptive. She is recently married and very concerned as she wants to conceive.

Which one of the following is the most appropriate next course of action?

- [ ] **A**   Arrange for a pelvic ultrasound
- [ ] **B**   Perform a pregnancy test
- [ ] **C**   Perform follicle-stimulating hormone (FSH) and luteinising hormone (LH levels)
- [ ] **D**   Perform thyroid function tests
- [ ] **E**   Review her in 2 months' time

ANSWERS

THEME: GYNAECOLOGICAL INVESTIGATIONS

11.1   **K**   **Transvaginal ultrasound of the pelvis, Pipelle biopsy and saline sonography**

Although you might think that any of options C, J, or K may be right, in the NHS setting this is the most appropriate answer. Most hospitals have these one-stop 'postmenopausal bleeding clinics' where the diagnostic procedures are performed on an outpatient basis. Sonohysterography is gradually replacing outpatient hysteroscopy as it can be combined with the scan to give a more detailed pelvic assessment. It is also more patient friendly. The most likely diagnosis in this case is endometrial polyp, which is common in women using combined hormone replacement therapy.

11.2   **E**   **Diagnostic laparotomy**

This is a scenario of ruptured ectopic pregnancy and E is the only possible answer. It is the only life-threatening gynaecological emergency that requires immediate surgery.

11.3   **D**   **Diagnostic laparoscopy and tubal dye test**

The symptoms described here by the patient point towards endometriosis. Although both transvaginal HyCoSy and HSG (hysterosalpingogram) help in diagnosing tubal and other uterine structural problems, they cannot assess the pelvis to diagnose endometriosis. Hence, it may be worthwhile to first think of the disease and then work out the best diagnostic modality in the given scenario.

11.4   I   Serum LH and serum FSH

This is because there is suspicion of premature ovarian failure based on the symptoms.

11.5   A   Cervical punch biopsy

This is obviously a case of suspected cervical malignancy that needs to be ruled out by tissue biopsy. As the patient is an asylum seeker it means she is not in the National Cervical Screening Programme.

THEME: CONTRACEPTION

11.6   C   Dianette

Dianette is the trade name for co-cyprindiol, which is a mixture of cyproterone acetate 2mg and ethinylestradiol 35 micrograms. This is an antiandrogen and reduces acne by decreasing the sebum secretion, which is under androgen control. Dianette is the only licensed drug for acne and hirsutism in the UK. It is ideal for people who need contraception and for whom acne is also a problem.

11.7   K   Progesterone-only pill

This does not affect the volume of breast milk and provides 99% contraceptive efficacy when breastfeeding. The lactational amenorrhoea method (LAM) cannot be considered when the mother is not fully breastfeeding. Women may be advised that if they are less than 6 months' postpartum, amenorrhoeic and fully breastfeeding (no other liquids or solids given), the LAM is over 98% effective in preventing pregnancy.

11.8   G   Intrauterine copper device

A copper intrauterine contraceptive device (IUCD) can be inserted up to 5 days following unprotected intercourse at any time in the menstrual cycle provided this is the only unprotected sex that has occurred since the last period. If there has been unprotected sex more than once since the last period then the IUCD can be fitted up to 5 days after the earliest time ovulation could have occurred (day 14 in a 28-day cycle).

The 'morning-after pill' is also known as 'post-coital contraception' and the recommended method is one dose of Levonelle (levonorgestrel 1500 μg) taken as soon as possible after unprotected intercourse. If taken within 24 hours it will prevent up to 95% of pregnancies, and up to 85% if taken between 24–48 hours. If taken between 49 and 72 hours it will prevent up to 58% of pregnancies. It is only licensed to be taken within 72 hours of unprotected intercourse, as the efficacy after this is unknown.

11.9   J   Mirena coil

Considering the patient's age, her high BMI and menstrual problems this seems the best option. The Mirena coil is a progesterone-only intrauterine system that releases 20 μg of levonorgestrel directly into the uterine cavity every 24 hours. It acts by preventing endometrial proliferation and is very effective in controlling menorrhagia.

11.10   E   Implanon

This patient has a problem with contraceptive compliance and needs reliable long-term contraception. Taking into consideration that she has had a sexually transmitted infection in the past, IUCD would not be ideal for her. Although you can consider condoms, her history of poor compliance with the pill and injections and also the poor efficacy of condoms will not make these an ideal choice for her. Implanon is an implant containing a progesterone contraceptive. It contains etonogestrel, is subdermally implanted and is effective for 3 years. It also has a very low Pearl Index (ie the measure of contraceptive efficacy expressed in 100 women-reproductive years). She should be advised that nuisance bleeding can occur, particularly in the first few months after insertion.

THEME: INFERTILITY/ASSISTED REPRODUCTIVE TECHNOLOGY

This is a difficult theme as infertility is not the forte of most people. It is important to try to identify whether it is the man, woman, or both, with the problem. Once you have done that then you can work out which is the best technique to overcome the problem.

11.11   F   IVF with ICSI

In this case there are both male (low count with poor motility) and female (poor quality eggs associated with an age of more than 35) factors involved, which are best overcome by this technique.

11.12   C   IUI

There is a male factor problem here. Hypospadias is a congenital defect where the urethra opens on the underside of the penis instead of the tip, hence there is an anatomical difficulty in the sperm reaching the egg. This can be overcome by IUI.

11.13   H   Ovulation induction with follicular tracking

This is the first-line medical management for women with anovulatory cycles. Some women with polycystic ovarian syndrome who are refractory to ovulation induction can opt for surgical management in the form of laparoscopic multiple-diathermy punctures of the ovary.

11.14   D   IVF

This is fairly straightforward as the absence of tubes rules out the other options such as GIFT/ZIFT. As the woman has conceived twice in the past, this rules out male subfertility.

11.15   I   Surrogacy

The patient, having had a hysterectomy, has lost her uterus and hence will be unable to bear any pregnancy. Thus they will need a donor uterus to bear their pregnancy, which can be provided by a surrogate mother. Once they have had a successful IVF cycle with the host egg and sperm, the embryos will then by transferred into the surrogate mother's uterus.

THEME: SEXUALLY TRANSMITTED INFECTIONS

11.16   A   Chancroid

Chancroid, or soft chancre, is an acute sexually transmitted infection, caused by *Haemophilus ducreyi*, which is endemic in parts of Asia and Africa. This is a painful chancre whereas syphilitic or lymphogranuloma venereum ulcers are painless.

11.17   G   Herpes simplex

Genital herpes is caused by the herpes simplex virus. In general type 1 is responsible for oral herpes or cold sores and type 2 for genital herpes. However, it is best if possible to culture the virus and obtain sensitivities, as there are now some strains resistant to aciclovir.

11.18   I   HIV

Oral candidiasis is one of the opportunistic infections found in immunosuppressed patients with HIV infection. Kaposi sarcoma is a cutaneous manifestation of acquired immune deficiency syndrome (AIDS), initially caused by proliferation of small blood vessels in the dermis. Later, nodules are formed with proliferating spindle cells and intradermal haemorrhage and the deposition of haemosiderin.

11.19   C   Gonorrhoea

The symptoms are classic of gonococcal pelvic inflammatory disease. The finding of a Bartholin abscess is diagnostic. In the past more than 50% of women in the reproductive age group with a Bartholin abscess tested positive for gonorrhoea but the level varies according to the type of population being studied.

11.20   E   Hepatitis B

The viral markers make the diagnosis easy. The presence of anti-HBe gives a picture of chronic hepatitis B infection. Both hepatitis B and C can be contracted by intravenous drug users.

THEME: VAGINAL DISCHARGE

11.21   K   Vulvovaginitis

This is the commonest gynaecological problem in the prepubertal age group. Due to low levels of oestrogen between birth and puberty, the vaginal mucosa is thin and alkaline, making it less resistant to bacteria. Management takes the form of reassuring anxious parents, maintaining good hygiene and wearing cotton undergarments.

11.22   A   Atrophic vaginitis

This is a classic presentation. The dry, thin, atrophic vaginal mucosa rubs against the undergarments and causes bleeding and staining.

11.23   C   Candidiasis

This is a typical picture of vulval candidiasis and can be treated with clotrimazole pessaries or vaginal cream, or with a single dose of fluconazole 150 mg orally. It is also important to treat the partner to prevent reinfection.

11.24   E   Ectropion

This is the commonest cause of a clear, non-itchy vaginal discharge. This is common among pill users as it induces the columnar epithelium to spread over the transformation zone of the cervix. Columnar epithelium is secretory.

11.25   J   *Trichomonas vaginalis* infection

This is a typical discharge found in these infections. On per speculum examination the cervix is seen to have multiple small haemorrhagic areas, which lead to the description 'strawberry cervix'. Metronidazole 400 mg, twice/thrice a day for 7 days is the treatment of choice. It is important to take swabs to check sensitivities, and to screen for other sexually transmitted infections. Partner notification is also important.

THEME: VULVAL DISORDERS

11.26   C   Carcinoma of the vulva

The presence of such a characteristic ulcer with lymphadenopathy is diagnostic of a cancerous lesion.

11.27   J   Varicose veins

Vulval varicosity is worsened in pregnancy due to the pressure of the gravid uterus obstructing venous drainage from the lower extremity.

11.28   F   Leucoplakia

The only sure way to differentiate this from lichen sclerosis is by tissue biopsy. On clinical examination lichen sclerosis initially appears purplish and then turns white, with a shiny, thin skin.

11.29   M   Vulval wart

Vulval warts are caused by the human papillomavirus (HPV). They become more florid in immunosuppressed conditions such as pregnancy. Certain serotypes have been implicated in cervical intraepithelial neoplasia and there is now a vaccine to prevent infection of these. The warts are sexually transmitted and both partners need to be treated if present in both.

11.30   H   Sebaceous cyst

This is a typical presentation and the patient is often referred by the GP with a diagnosis of Bartholin abscess.

11.31   L   Vulval psoriasis

Psoriasis at this site is usually not scaly but still has the sharp demarcated edge of plaque psoriasis elsewhere. In candidiasis usually there are satellite lesions and in tinea cruris the margins are scaly and there is central clearing.

THEME: BREAST DISORDERS

11.32   G   Fibroadenoma

These are no longer thought to be benign breast tumours and are instead regarded as aberrations in breast development. However, you still need to investigate and reach your diagnosis based on a combination of scan and fine-needle aspiration cytology findings. Breast cysts usually occur after the age of 35 years.

11.33   D   Breast cancer

This is clearly a case of breast cancer. Skin dimpling is caused by local infiltration of malignancy and the peau d'orange appearance is due to lymphatic oedema. Both these signs are suggestive of locally advanced cancer.

11.34 E Duct ectasia

This condition is age-related and as women age the ducts shorten and dilate, resulting in inversion of the nipple. This should be differentiated from that seen in malignant conditions where the nipple appears retracted and pulled in.

11.35 C Breast abscess

The mention of swelling clearly helps in making the diagnosis. Non-lactational breast abscesses are becoming more common and the causative organisms are usually *Staphylococcus* and/or other anaerobes.

11.36 J Lipoma

These are benign fatty lumps that occur in any part of the body where fat can expand.

11.37 E Increase in total lung capacity

Total lung capacity is decreased in pregnancy by about 200 ml. This is because the residual volume is reduced by 200 ml, secondary to the large intra-abdominal swelling in pregnancy.

11.38 D Day 21 progesterone level

This is the easiest test to check the ovulatory status. If D21 progesterone results are more than 30 nmol/l in two cycles, the woman is ovulating.

11.39 B The fetus will probably be harmed

Intrahepatic cholestasis of pregnancy is associated with increased fetal loss. Recurrent cholestasis may occur during subsequent pregnancies.

11.40   B   Perform a pregnancy test

If the patient has not done a pregnancy test then this needs to be done first. Secondary amenorrhoea is due to pregnancy until proved otherwise. Even denial of sexual activity should be taken with a degree of circumspection. 'Post-pill amenorrhoea' is when stopping oral contraceptives does not lead to a resumption of a normal menstrual cycle. It usually settles spontaneously in about 3 months but if not it will need to be investigated. The condition is probably not a true entity as the cause of amenorrhoea started while taking the contraceptives. These induced an artificial cycle until they were stopped.

Chapter 12
Respiratory

QUESTIONS

THEME: MANAGEMENT OF OBSTRUCTIVE AIRWAYS DISEASES

Options

A Combination of salmeterol and fluticasone

B Fluticasone

C Ipratropium nebuliser

D Long-term oxygen therapy

E Magnesium sulphate

F Salbutamol nebuliser

G Salmeterol

H Terbutaline inhaler

I Theophylline tablets

J Tiotropium

K Zafirlukast tablets

For each of the patients below, choose the single most appropriate agent from the list of options above. Each option may be used once, more than once or not at all.

☐ **12.1** **A patient presents with severe chronic obstructive pulmonary disease (COPD), a forced expiratory volume in one second (FEV$_1$) of 0.8 litres and three hospital admissions in the past year. For which agent is there enough evidence showing that it will reduce the rate of acute exacerbation and improve quality of life with no impact on pulmonary function?**

☐ **12.2** A patient with moderate COPD and an FEV$_1$ of 1.5 litres has been admitted to hospital twice this year (one admission last year). He already uses a salbutamol inhaler as required, an ipratropium inhaler four times per day and a combination of a steroid and a long-acting β-agonist inhaler. Which agent should be introduced after stopping one of his medications?

☐ **12.3** A 58-year-old man has severe COPD. Arterial blood gases on air when he was well showed pH 7.36 (normal 7.36–7.44), $p(O_2)$ 7.2 kPa (normal 11–13 kPa) and $p(CO_2)$ 6.6 kPa (normal 4.7–5.9 kPa). An echocardiogram showed right ventricular dilatation and dysfunction. Which is the only agent known to improve morbidity and mortality?

☐ **12.4** A 45-year-old woman with brittle asthma, using a salbutamol inhaler prn and a combination steroid and salmeterol inhaler, is experiencing acute flare-ups necessitating recurrent hospital admission. Which would be the next agent to introduce?

☐ **12.5** A 42-year-old woman with known asthma uses a salbutamol inhaler 200 μg when needed and beclometasone 400 μg/day. She has recurrent episodes of disturbed sleep, cough and shortness of breath. Which would be the next agent to introduce?

☐ **12.6** A 26-year-old man arrives in accident and emergency with acute severe asthma. His peak flow measured in the ambulance was 48% of predicted, and he has had nebulised salbutamol, 40 mg oral prednisolone and high-flow oxygen. He has not responded well. He is given another nebuliser, this time a combination of salbutamol and ipratropium, but he is becoming exhausted and his oxygen saturation is now 91%. Which agent should be used next?

THEME: PNEUMONIA

Options

A Cytomegalovirus
B *Klebsiella pneumoniae*
C *Legionella pneumophila*
D *Mycoplasma pneumoniae*
E *Pneumocystis jiroveci*
F *Pseudomonas aeruginosa*
G Streptococcal pneumonia
H Tuberculosis

For each of the patients below, choose the single most appropriate answer from the list of options above. Each option may be used once, more than once or not at all.

☐ **12.7** A 56-year-old man with no underlying lung problems went on holiday to Cyprus. He developed a dry cough and cold, which seemed like a viral prodromal illness. After 4–5 days he felt confused and started with diarrhoea and vomiting. A blood test shows a white blood cell count of 11.6 x 10⁹/l, neutrophils 10.1 x 10⁹/l, lymphocytes 0.7 x 10⁹/l, eosinophils 0.3 x 10⁹/l, monocytes 0.5 x 10⁹/l. He is also found to have hyponatraemia, hypoalbuminaemia and a high level of aspartate aminotransferase (AST).

☐ **12.8** A 70-year-old woman with known chronic obstructive pulmonary disease and diabetes presents with increased shortness of breath, some streaky haemoptysis and a cough that produces purulent green sputum. She is also a known alcoholic. Her chest X-ray revealed extensive bilateral consolidation.

☐ **12.9** A 22-year-old man with known cystic fibrosis presents with a cough and breathlessness, which are much worse than usual.

☐ **12.10** A 16-year-old boy living in an institution presents with headache and malaise that preceded a dry cough by 48 hours. He has also developed a rash, predominantly on his arms and legs. Blood tests show his haemoglobin to be 10.1 g/dl, with a reticulocyte count of 5% and thrombocytopenia. His chest X-ray shows bilateral extensive shadowing in both lungs.

☐ **12.11** A 58-year-old renal transplant recipient who is on ciclosporin has developed a high fever, severe breathlessness and a dry cough. His chest X-ray shows mild shadowing in the perihilar region on the right side. Pulse oximetry demonstrates gross desaturation on air.

THEME: DISEASES OF THE RESPIRATORY SYSTEM

Options

A   Ankylosing spondylitis

B   Churg–Strauss syndrome

C   Cryptogenic organising pneumonia

D   Extrinsic allergic alveolitis

E   Goodpasture syndrome

F   Motor neurone disease

G   Progressive massive fibrosis (PMF)

H   Tropical pulmonary eosinophilia

For each of the patients below, choose the single most appropriate answer from the list of options above. Each option may be used once, more than once or not at all.

☐ **12.12**   A non-smoker who had worked in coal pits for 20 years presents with gradually increasing shortness of breath, limited exercise tolerance and a dry cough. His chest X-ray shows round fibrotic masses in the upper lobes with central cavitation. Lung function testing demonstrates a mixed restrictive and obstructive ventilatory defect with irreversible airflow limitation and reduced gas transfer.

☐ **12.13**   A 56-year-old man presents with breathlessness, which predominantly occurs when he is supine. He also has symptoms of sleep apnoea and daytime headaches and somnolence. Spirometry shows a decreased tidal volume and vital capacity.

☐ **12.14**   A 35-year-old man has received a diagnosis of allergic rhinitis and asthma. Examination revealed a peripheral neuropathy with tingling and numbness in a glove and stocking distribution. Skin lesions are present in the form of tender subcutaneous nodules. The patient is responding well to corticosteroids.

☐ **12.15** A 48-year-old farmer presented with fever, malaise, cough and shortness of breath. He also complains of severe weight loss. On examination he is cyanosed, and tachypnoeic with coarse and inspiratory crackles and wheeze throughout his chest. His chest X-ray shows fluffy nodular shadowing and there is a polymorphonuclear leucocytosis.

THEME: BLOOD GAS ANALYSIS

Options

A Diabetes

B Head injury

C Mild asthma

D Paracetamol poisoning

E Primary hyperventilation

F Pulmonary embolism

G Severe asthma

H Tension pneumothorax

For each of the following blood gas results, select the single most likely diagnosis from the list of options above. Each option may be used once, more than once or not at all.

☐ **12.16**	pH 6.91	$p(CO_2)$ 2.6	$p(O_2)$ 15.7	Base excess –22
☐ **12.17**	pH 7.52	$p(CO_2)$ 2.6	$p(O_2)$ 15.7	Base excess +2
☐ **12.18**	pH 7.37	$p(CO_2)$ 2.6	$p(O_2)$ 9.4	Base excess +2
☐ **12.19**	pH 7.21	$p(CO_2)$ 7.4	$p(O_2)$ 8.4	Base excess +8
Normal values				
	pH 7.36–7.44	$p(CO_2)$ 4.7–5.9 kPa	$p(O_2)$ 11–13 kPa	Base excess –2 – +2 mmol/l.

THEME: CAUSES OF RESPIRATORY SYMPTOMS IN CHILDREN

Options

A   Acute bronchiolitis

B   Allergic rhinitis

C   Asthma

D   Congenital cardiac disease

E   Croup

F   Cystic fibrosis

G   Diphtheria

H   Epiglottitis

I   Inhaled foreign body

J   Pneumonia

K   Respiratory distress syndrome

L   Tracheo-oesophageal fistula

M   Whooping cough

For each of the patients below, choose the single most likely diagnosis from the list of options above. Each option may be used once, more than once or not at all.

☐ **12.20 A 3-year-old boy has had a chronic cough for 3 months. He has had several chest infections and has required several courses of antibiotics. On examination a monophonic wheeze is heard in the right lower lung field. He is systemically well.**

☐ **12.21 A 6-year-old refugee from Chechnya is unwell with a high fever, sore throat and harsh cough. She has some difficulty swallowing and has a hoarse voice. There is a thick grey exudate on the tonsils.**

☐ **12.22** A 1-month-old baby has had a chronic cough since birth and has been treated for two episodes of pneumonia. He becomes cyanosed when feeding. He is on the third centile for weight. When coughing, he produces copious amounts of secretions and appears to 'blow bubbles'.

☐ **12.23** A 3-year-old girl has had a paroxysmal nocturnal cough intermittently for the past 6–8 months. She is well during the day with only a tendency to cough on exertion. The mother complains that each time she gets a cold 'it goes to her chest' and she has had frequent antibiotic treatment. There is a history of mild eczema. Clinically, except for dry skin no abnormalities are noted.

☐ **12.24** An 18-month-old has had a paroxysmal nocturnal cough associated with a 'persistent cold' that has not cleared for several weeks. She starts to cough as she goes to sleep and may retch and vomit on some occasions. The cough is not severe during the day but she sounds 'rattly'. There is a strong history of atopy in the family.

THEME: ALLERGIC LUNG DISEASE

Options

A   Berylliosis

B   Byssinosis

C   Churg-Strauss

D   Extrinsic allergic alveolitis

E   Pneumoconiosis

F   Siderosis

For each of the patients described below, choose the single most appropriate answer from the list of options above. Each option may be used once, more than once or not at all.

☐ **12.25** A 53-year-old welder presents with mild cough and shortness of breath. The chest X-ray shows dense nodular shadowing.

☐ **12.26** A 45-year-old weaver presents with chest tightness, cough and shortness of breath, which improve at the weekends. The chest X-ray is normal.

☐ **12.27** A 60-year-old smoker who was made redundant from his coal mining job in the 1980s presents with exertional dyspnoea and cough. He has a mixed restrictive and obstructive pattern on spirometry. The chest X-ray shows round fibrotic masses in the upper lobes.

☐ **12.28** A 56-year-old stonemason presents with dry cough and nail splitting.

☐ **12.29** A 45-year-old farmer presents with flu-like symptoms and cough which occur every autumn.

12.30 A 45-year-old smoker of 20 pack-years has incidentally been found on X-ray to have a tumour in his right lung.

Which one of the following statements about investigation of this condition is not true?

☐ **A** Bilateral lymphangitis carcinomatosa on chest X-ray is more often indicative of a primary tumour in the lung

☐ **B** Breath scan has about 85% specificity in predicting lung cancer without histology

☐ **C** Computed tomography (CT)-guided, fine-needle aspiration is associated with pneumothorax in 25% of cases

☐ **D** Magnetic resonance imaging (MRI) is more effective than a CT scan in the staging of lung cancer

☐ **E** Spirometry, especially forced expiratory volume in one second (FEV_1), is necessary to decide the appropriateness of surgery

12.31 A 52-year-old man is diagnosed as having obstructive sleep apnoea (OSA) syndrome.

Which one of the following statements about the management of his condition is true?

☐ **A** Acetazolamide is considered to be an effective treatment in mild to moderate OSA

☐ **B** Continuous positive airway pressure (CPAP) is useful only in OSA and not in central sleep apnoea

☐ **C** In patients with ischaemic heart disease and OSA, nasal CPAP is considered the treatment of choice

☐ **D** Intraoral devices are effective in a minority of patients

☐ **E** Uvulopalatopharyngoplasty is effective in more than 90% of patients with OSA

12.32 A 3-year-old child presents with a 3-month history of recurrent episodes of cough and wheeze. The cough is worse at night. Chest examination is normal between episodes of wheeze, but there is prolonged expiratory wheeze during an episode.

Which one of the following is the most appropriate management?

- ☐ **A** Arrange chest X-ray
- ☐ **B** Full blood count
- ☐ **C** Treat with a course of antibiotics
- ☐ **D** Trial of antihistaminics
- ☐ **E** Trial of bronchodilators

ANSWERS

THEME: MANAGEMENT OF OBSTRUCTIVE AIRWAYS DISEASES

12.1   B   Fluticasone

The British Thoracic Society (BTS) guidelines and the National Institute for Health and Clinical Excellence (NICE) guidelines recommend the use of steroid inhalers in patients with severe COPD and repeated hospitalisations, irrespective of lung function parameters.

12.2   J   Tiotropium

Tiotropium, a long-acting anticholinergic agent, brings about a marked improvement in quality of life and reduces the number of hospital admissions for patients with moderate to severe COPD. It cannot, however, be used in conjunction with ipratropium.

12.3   D   Long-term oxygen therapy

Oxygen is the only agent that has been shown to improve survival in patients with severe COPD and cor pulmonale.

12.4   K   Zafirlukast

The BTS guidelines (www.brit-thoracic.org.uk/Guidelinessince%201997_ asthma_html) recommend introducing a leukotriene antagonist at 'Step 3' of management where treatment with long-acting beta agonists (LABA) has failed to produce any response, or at 'Step 4' where despite a response to maximal LABA and steroid treatment the patient has persistent inadequate control.

12.5   G   Salmeterol

Salmeterol has been shown to be very effective in controlling the disturbed sleep in people with asthma. It acts better when used in conjunction with a steroid inhaler.

12.6   E   Magnesium sulphate

Patients with severe asthma may be helped by magnesium sulphate (unlicensed indication) but evidence of benefit is limited. It may be given as an iv infusion or by nebulisation.

THEME: PNEUMONIA

12.7   C   *Legionella pneumophila*

A strong presumptive diagnosis of legionella is possible in the majority of patients when three of the following four features are present: a prodromal viral illness; a dry cough, confusion or diarrhoea; lymphopenia without marked leucocytosis; and hyponatraemia.

12.8   B   *Klebsiella pneumoniae*

Pneumonia occurs in elderly patients who have a pre-existing comorbidity such as diabetes and alcoholism. Upper lobe cavitating lesions are common with bulging of the fissures. This organism can be found in sputum and in blood cultures.

12.9   F   *Pseudomonas aeruginosa*

The presence of this organism correlates with a worsening clinical condition and higher mortality in patients with cystic fibrosis. It is important to culture the sputum, as this organism is resistant to most of the common antibiotics used to treat pneumonia.

12.10   D   *Mycoplasma pneumoniae*

Infection with this organism may result in cough and dramatic X-ray appearances, which may last for weeks. Patients can have a relapse. Extrapulmonary complications such as pericarditis, haemolytic anaemia, Stevens–Johnson syndrome and neurological problems are rare. Exanthems can also occur.

12.11   E   *Pneumocystis jiroveci* (formerly known as *Pneumocystis carinii*)

In contrast to infection with mycoplasma, the clinical features of *Pneumocystis jiroveci* pneumonia are far worse than the radiological appearances. In 90% of cases the diagnosis can be made by using indirect immunofluorescence with monoclonal antibodies to stain sputum.

THEME: DISEASES OF THE RESPIRATORY SYSTEM

12.12   G   Progressive massive fibrosis

PMF occurs in 30% of patients with a background of category 3 simple pneumoconiosis. They have considerable effort dyspnoea, which may progress even after exposure to coal dust has ceased.

12.13   F   Motor neurone disease

Any cause of bilateral diaphragmatic weakness or paralysis causes a decrease in tidal volume and an increased respiratory rate. Sniffing causes a paradoxical inward movement of the abdominal wall, best seen in the supine position.

CHAPTER 12 ANSWERS

12.14   B   Churg–Strauss syndrome

This syndrome presents with a triad of rhinitis and asthma, eosinophilia and systemic vasculitis. It typically involves the lungs, peripheral nerves and skin, but spares the kidneys. The disease responds well to corticosteroid treatment.

12.15   D   Extrinsic allergic alveolitis

Continued exposure will lead to features of fibrosing alveolitis. Prevention is the aim. Prednisolone in high doses will lead to the regression of the disease in the early stages.

THEME: BLOOD GAS ANALYSIS

12.16   A   Diabetes

A base excess more negative than –2 indicates metabolic acidosis as in this case. A base excess more positive than +2 indicates metabolic alkalosis. This patient is hyperventilating to compensate for the metabolic acidosis. Diabetic ketoacidosis would be the commonest cause.

12.17   E   Primary hyperventilation

This patient is also hyperventilating, which has pushed the blood oxygen above normal and made him mildly alkalotic. There is no hypoxia or metabolic acidosis so no evident reason for the hyperventilation.

12.18   F   Pulmonary embolism

This patient is also hyperventilating but is still hypoxic. This implies a problem with gas exchange in the lungs and an increased ventilation/ perfusion ratio mismatch. Pneumonia would be a common cause, but a normal chest X-ray would make pulmonary embolism the likely cause.

12.19   G   Severe asthma

In a moderate asthma attack, the carbon dioxide is low as the patient hyperventilates; as the patient deteriorates and tires the carbon dioxide becomes normal and then raised. This patient is in danger of respiratory arrest.

THEME: CAUSES OF RESPIRATORY SYMPTOMS IN CHILDREN

12.20   I   Inhaled foreign body

Cough with wheeze is most often due to asthma. Localised, monophonic (single-pitched) wheeze suggests obstruction of a single airway. A common cause in young children is inhalation of a foreign body, often without any history to confirm this. Inhaled foreign objects are most likely to become trapped in the bronchus to the right lower lobe. A chest X-ray often makes the diagnosis. Otherwise diagnosis and treatment is with bronchoscopy.

12.21   G   Diphtheria

Diphtheria has almost been eradicated from the UK. However, political turmoil and increasing poverty in eastern Europe and the former Soviet states have caused a massive increase in diphtheria. It is highly infectious so early identification and contact tracing is important. Diagnosis should be suspected clinically by the presence of a fever and adherent membrane over the tonsils, palate or uvula. Tachycardia, out of proportion to the degree of fever, suggests myocarditis, which may be irreversible or fatal. Diagnose with culture of a throat swab. Treat early with diphtheria antitoxin and penicillin or erythromycin.

12.22   L   Tracheo-oesophageal fistula

Oesophageal atresia and tracheo-oesophageal fistulae may present immediately after birth with inability to feed. They may also present with failure to thrive, nasal regurgitation, recurrent aspiration pneumonia, cough or cyanosis.

12.23   C   Asthma

Asthma in childhood presents with varying grades of severity. It may present with persistent cough with no history of wheezing, which may occur mainly at night or with exercise. The other common trigger in childhood is viral upper respiratory infections that are treated as 'chest infections' with repeated courses of antibiotics. There will be a history of atopy in the family in many instances.

12.24   B   Allergic rhinitis

A child with a 'persistent cold' is most likely to have allergic (perennial) rhinitis. The child has nasal obstruction due to mucosal oedema and has a persistent thin mucoid discharge which causes a postnasal drip leading to paroxysmal cough especially at night. The cough could be severe enough to cause vomiting and retching. The constant production of the secretions lead to the noisy breathing and a rattly chest mistakenly treated as asthma.

THEME: ALLERGIC LUNG DISEASE

12.25   F   Siderosis

This is caused by reaction to iron dust. The chest X-ray findings are vastly out of proportion to the symptoms.

12.26 B   Byssinosis

This is an allergic reaction to cotton dust. The chest X-ray is generally normal. The symptoms are classically worst on Mondays, wane through the week and disappear when away from work.

12.27 E   Pneumoconiosis

12.28 E   Pneumoconiosis

Pneumoconiosis defines the process of accumulation of dust (often related to occupational exposure) in the lungs, which is permanent and may result in progressive tissue reaction. The condition may progress for many years after initial exposure, and may present with symptoms only after the exposure has ceased. A coal miner would have carbon deposits and a stonemason, silicon (silicosis).

12.29 D   Extrinsic allergic alveolitis

Farmer's lung is an example of extrinsic allergic alveolitis or hypersensitivity pneumonitis which is caused by hypersensitivity to the bacterium *Actinomycetes,* found on mouldy hay. It often worsens during the autumn when the hay is damp and allergens are found in high concentrations. Lung function tests reveal a restrictive pattern. The chest X-ray typically shows a nodular ground glass appearance. In the acute form, symptoms may completely resolve after exposure is removed.

12.30 A   Bilateral lymphangitis carcinomatosa on chest X-ray is more often indicative of a primary tumour in the lung

Bilateral lymphangitis carcinomatosa is more often associated with below-diaphragm primaries, eg stomach and colon.

12.31   **C**   **In patients with ischaemic heart disease and OSA, nasal CPAP is considered the treatment of choice**

Chronic OSA is associated with progressive right heart failure, respiratory acidosis and metabolic alkalosis. Carbonic anhydrase inhibitors, including acetazolamide, can minimise the metabolic consequences associated with sleep apnoea, but are only partially effective and reserved for those with severe metabolic derangement. CPAP is effective in reducing hypercapnia and improving oxygenation, and slows the progression to right heart failure. Weight loss, where appropriate, and intraoral and intranasal devices are usually sufficient for early management of patients with mild OSA. Uvulopalatopharyngoplasty is effective in a small minority of patients, and is performed only in selected patients with severe OSA.

12.32   **E**   **Trial of bronchodilators**

Usually the diagnosis of asthma is clear from the history and examination (including lung fraction testing), and investigation is not needed. Although a chest X-ray will often show hyperinflation, it will rarely influence management (but an X-ray is helpful for excluding congenital anomalies). Children over the age of 5 years can use a peak-flow meter, but under this age it is difficult to make a definitive diagnosis and often a trial of inhalers is used.

Mock Exam

Chapter 13
Clinical Problem Solving – Example Test Paper

QUESTIONS

Total time allowed is 90 minutes

THEME: HYPERTENSION TREATMENT

Options

A Amlodipine

B Atenolol

C Bendroflumethiazide

D Doxazosin

E Lisinopril

F Losartan

G Methyl dopa

H Moxonidine

For each of the hypertensive patients below, choose the single most likely antihypertensive medication from the list of options above. Each option may be used once, more than once or not at all.

☐ **13.1** A 60-year-old man with diabetes who is already taking an angiotensin-converting enzyme (ACE) inhibitor.

☐ **13.2** A 42-year-old African Caribbean woman with hypertension which is not controlled by bendroflumethiazide.

☐ **13.3** A 72-year-old man with poorly controlled hypertension who has recently developed angina.

☐ **13.4** A 41-year-old-woman with chronic obstructive pulmonary disease who is taking ramipril and bendroflumethiazide but has developed a persistent dry cough which does not seem to be related to her airways disease.

☐ **13.5** A 35-year-old pregnant woman whose blood pressure is 170/110 mmHg in the mid-trimester.

THEME: INFECTIOUS DISEASES IN CHILDHOOD

Options

A Intravenous aciclovir

B Intravenous antibiotic

C Oral aciclovir

D Oral antibiotic

E Symptomatic relief (antipyretics and/or analgesics)

F Topical aciclovir

G Topical antibiotic

For each of the patients below, choose the single most appropriate management option from the list of options above. Each option may be used once, more than once or not at all.

☐ **13.6** A 14-year-old girl has a 10-day history of fever and malaise. On examination there is prominent cervical lymphadenopathy.

☐ **13.7** A previously well 4-year-old girl has a fever and vesicular rash. It started as a papular rash on the trunk and spread peripherally with new spots appearing in crops.

☐ **13.8** A 10-month-old baby boy has fever and a widespread tender erythematous rash. The infant looks unwell and the skin is peeling in places.

☐ **13.9** A 3-year-old girl has multiple painful erosions on the mucosa of the mouth and tongue with erythema and swelling of the gums.

☐ **13.10** A 6-month-old baby boy has bilateral red eyes. There is a creamy sticky exudate in both eyes.

THEME: CHEST PAIN

Options

A   Acute angina

B   Bronchial carcinoma

C   Chest infection

D   Musculoskeletal pain

E   Myocardial infarction

F   Oesophageal reflux

G   Pulmonary embolism

H   Spontaneous pneumothorax

I   Unstable angina

For each of the patients below, choose the single most likely diagnosis from the list of options above. Each option may be used once, more than once or not at all.

☐ **13.11 A 62-year-old woman with chronic obstructive pulmonary disease presents with increasing wheeze and cough. Her inhalers are not working well and she has been coughing up purulent sputum. Her chest pain is much worse on deep inspiration and she has a slight fever.**

☐ **13.12 A 32-year-old woman presents with worsening shortness of breath and pain on deep inspiration. She had her first baby 2 weeks ago and is usually fit and well.**

☐ **13.13 A 52-year-old builder smokes 25 cigarettes a day. He has worsening left-sided chest pain which does not radiate and he can point one finger to the site of the pain. It has been present for 2 days and he is usually fit and well.**

☐ **13.14** A 73-year-old woman has coronary heart disease. She takes aspirin, atenolol and ramipril. The past 3 nights she has been awoken in the night with left-sided chest pain radiating down her left arm. She has tried her glyceryl trinitrate spray but without effect, the pain passing off eventually after about half an hour.

☐ **13.15** A 56-year-old bricklayer presents with central chest pain for 2 days. It is not related to exertion. He has been working overtime recently and taking regular ibuprofen for a sprained wrist.

THEME: FACIAL RASHES

Options

A Acne vulgaris

B Actinic keratoses

C Erysipelas

D Perioral dermatitis

E Psoriasis

F Rosacea

G Seborrhoeic eczema

H Sunburn

I Systemic lupus erythematosus

For each of the patients below, choose the single most likely diagnosis from the list of options above. Each option may be used once, more than once or not at all.

☐ **13.16** A 13-year-old girl has papules and comedones on her chin and forehead. She cleanses her face twice a day. She has recently started her periods.

☐ **13.17** A 70-year-old man has erythematous macules and papules with coarse adherent scale on his forehead and bald scalp. Many of the lesions have become confluent.

☐ **13.18** A 30-year-old woman has papules and erythema around the mouth and on her chin. Her son's topical steroid helped but the rash became much worse when she stopped using it.

☐ **13.19** A 65-year-old woman has a persistent erythematous eruption on her forehead and cheeks. It has become much worse after her summer holiday to Italy. There are a few pustules within it.

☐ **13.20** A 45-year-old man has had dandruff for many years. He has greasy, red and scaly skin on his central face and forehead. The sides of his nose down to the outer ends of his mouth are also affected.

THEME: MACROSCOPIC HAEMATURIA

Options

A   Bladder cancer

B   Glomerulonephritis

C   Haemorrhagic cystitis (urinary infection)

D   Prostate cancer

E   Prostatitis

F   Renal cancer

G   Renal cyst

H   Schistosomiasis

I   Sickle cell disease

J   Ureteric calculus

For each of the patients below, choose the single most likely diagnosis from the list of options above. Each option may be used once, more than once or not at all.

☐ **13.21   A partially sighted 80-year-old woman has a fractured humerus after a trivial injury. She is catheterised and found to have macroscopic haematuria.**

☐ **13.22   A 50-year-old man has terminal uralgia, frequency and haematuria. Urine culture does not reveal any organisms.**

☐ **13.23   A 20-year-old male visitor from Egypt has severe frequency and dysuria and has seen blood in the urine.**

☐ **13.24   A 70-year-old woman has recently started taking warfarin for atrial fibrillation. She feels well but notices blood in the urine.**

☐ **13.25   A 90-year-old woman in a nursing home uses pads for urinary incontinence. She is already taking antibiotics for a urinary infection, has new-onset confusion and now frank haematuria.**

THEME: SHORT STATURE IN CHILDREN

Options

A   Achondroplasia

B   Congenital hypothyroidism

C   Down syndrome

D   Growth hormone deficiency

E   Klinefelter syndrome

F   Noonan syndrome

G   Russell–Silver syndrome

H   Turner syndrome

For each of the children below, choose the most likely cause of short stature from the list of options above. Each option may be used once, more than once or not at all.

☐ **13.26** A child with an abnormally sized head and predominant shortening of the proximal upper and lower limbs.

☐ **13.27** A 6-year-old boy with webbing of the neck, cubitus valgus and congenital heart disease.

☐ **13.28** A 7-year-old boy previously treated with cranial irradiation for a brain tumour has recurrent episodes of hypoglycaemia.

☐ **13.29** A 2-year-old with poor motor and speech development, large tongue and umbilical hernia.

THEME: CAUSES OF A NON-BLANCHING RASH

Options

A Acute leukaemia

B Cushing disease

C Fat embolism syndrome

D Haemolytic–uraemic syndrome

E Henoch–Schönlein purpura

F Immune thrombocytopenic purpura

G Meningococcal septicaemia

H Non-accidental injury

For each of the following descriptions, choose the single most likely diagnosis from the list of options above. Each option may be used once, more than once or not at all.

☐ **13.30** A child with malaise and a mild fever presents with a purpuric rash on the buttocks and legs. Otherwise he is well.

☐ **13.31** Following a recent upper respiratory tract infection, a previously well child has started to bruise easily. Their platelet count is 10 x 10^9/l.

☐ **13.32** A child presents with four lines of purpura along the outer thigh. The platelet count is 200 x 10^9/l.

☐ **13.33** A very sick child with high fever, has a purpuric rash on the limbs and a prolonged capillary refill time.

☐ **13.34** A 6-year-old child has developed widespread petechiae and is pale. She has been unwell for a few weeks with recurrent infections.

THEME: INVESTIGATIONS OF PRURITUS VULVAE

Options

A Creatinine clearance

B Glucose tolerance test

C High vaginal swab

D Vulval biopsy

E None of the above

For each presentation of pruritus vulvae below, choose the single most appropriate investigation from the list above. Each option may be used once, more than once or not at all.

☐ **13.35** A woman with associated history of vaginal discharge.

☐ **13.36** A woman with a history of postmenopausal bleeding.

☐ **13.37** This investigation is unnecessary in pruritus vulvae.

☐ **13.38** A 45-year-old woman with associated vulval ulceration.

☐ **13.39** In a 50-year-old obese woman with features of candidiasis.

THEME: CAUSES OF CLUBBING

Options

A   Axillary artery aneurysm

B   Bronchiectasis

C   Coeliac disease

D   Crohn disease

E   Cyanotic congenital heart disease

F   Cystic fibrosis

G   Fibrosing alveolitis

H   Hepatic cirrhosis

I   Hyperthyroidism

J   Infective endocarditis

K   Mesothelioma

L   Squamous cell lung cancer

For each patient below, choose the most likely cause of clubbing from the list of options above. Each option may be used once, more than once or not at all.

☐ **13.40** A 74-year-old man has fever and breathlessness. He recently had a transurethral resection of the prostate but was otherwise well until 3 weeks ago. His temperature is 37.7°C, his pulse is 96/min and regular, and his blood pressure is 180/80 mmHg. He has an early diastolic murmur. His chest is clear. Blood is seen on urine dipstick test. He has evidence of early clubbing.

☐ **13.41** A 27-year-old woman has recurrent chest infections and has a chronic productive cough. She remembers having had whooping cough as a child. She is not febrile or cyanosed but has marked clubbing. She has widespread crackles and a wheeze which do not clear with coughing.

☐ **13.42** A 68-year-old man has a 3-month history of cough and weight loss. He is cachectic and has a hyperexpanded, quiet chest with no abnormal breath sounds heard. He has left-sided ptosis and bilateral clubbing. He recently stopped smoking and gives a history of asbestos exposure.

☐ **13.43** A 15-year-old boy is under investigation for weight loss. He has intermittent abdominal pain and diarrhoea. His stools are often pale and hard to flush away. He is thin and pale-skinned with fair hair but with no specific abnormalities apart from clubbing.

☐ **13.44** A 53-year-old man has clubbing in the left hand only. He has hypertension and angina, with three-vessel coronary disease shown on angiography 2 years ago. His hypertension and angina are well controlled.

THEME: COMMON PRESENTATIONS OF SPORTSMEN/WOMEN

Options

A Anterior knee pain

B Bucket handle meniscus tear

C Carpal tunnel syndrome

D Lateral epicondylitis

E Plantar fasciitis

F Prepatellar bursitis

G Pulled elbow

H Shin splints

I Trochanteric bursitis

J Ulnar collateral ligament rupture

For each of the presentations below, choose the single most appropriate answer from the list above. Each option may be used once, more than once or not at all.

☐ **13.45** A skier consults after a fall in which he was not seriously injured. He fell doing slalom while holding his ski poles and now has pain.

☐ **13.46** An amateur runner is trying to train for the London Marathon.

☐ **13.47** A professional violin player presents with pain during rehearsals.

☐ **13.48** A footballer has fallen during a tackle.

☐ **13.49** A female competitive rower complains of pain.

THEME: HEADACHE

Options

A Brain tumour

B Cluster headache

C Migraine

D Subarachnoid haemorrhage

E Temporal arteritis

F Tension headache

E Trigeminal neuralgia

For each of the patients below, choose the single most likely diagnosis from the list of options above. Each option may be used once, more than once or not at all.

☐ **13.50** A 33-year-old housewife comes to your surgery complaining of worsening headache over 24 hours. This has been associated with nausea and some photophobia. That morning, before the headache started, she saw some zig-zag lines and felt unwell. She is otherwise well and only takes an oral contraceptive pill.

☐ **13.51** A 42-year-old man complains of recurrent headaches on the left side of his head. The pain comes on very rapidly and sometimes when he has the headache his left eye becomes watery and bloodshot. He is a smoker.

☐ **13.52** A 48-year-old man has a worsening headache at the back of his head. He has recently changed jobs and been under a lot of stress. He says the headache came on suddenly during the night and woke him from his sleep. He also has some photophobia.

☐ **13.53** A 70-year-old man describes a sharp, intermittent pain on the left side of his face. It often comes on when he is shaving or eating. The pain lasts a couple of minutes. He says it is very severe.

☐ **13.54** A 45-year-old nurse complains of worsening headache. She describes it like a band across her forehead, sometimes worse on the left side. It worsens throughout the day. Simple analgesics are ineffective and she is worried she may have a brain tumour.

☐ **13.55** A 67-year-old man complains of a worsening, severe headache which is often aggravated by combing his hair. He has been feeling more tired than usual.

THEME: FAILURE TO CONCEIVE

Options

A   Endocervical and high vaginal swab

B   Hysterosalpingogram

C   Karyotype analysis

D   Pelvic ultrasound scan

E   Serum luteinising hormone (LH) and follicle-stimulating hormone (FSH)

F   Serum prolactin

G   Serum testosterone

For each of the scenarios described below, choose the single most appropriate initial investigation from the list of options above. Each option may be used once, more than once or not at all.

☐ **13.56** A 26-year-old has failed to conceive after one year. Her periods are regular. She has normal secondary sexual characteristics. Pelvic examination reveals right adnexal tenderness. She admits to several 'one night stands' in the past although she is currently in a steady relationship.

☐ **13.57** A 30-year-old has been trying to conceive for 18 months. She has irregular periods which can be anything from 2–6 weeks apart, and she also had acne in her early 20s. On examination she is slightly overweight, but there are no other remarkable findings. LH and FSH are within the normal range.

☐ **13.58** A 44-year-old would like to become pregnant. She was recently married and is keen to start a family as quickly as possible. Her periods used to be regular but recently have been more infrequent, at intervals of 6–8 weeks.

☐ **13.59** An 18-year-old woman presents with primary amenorrhoea. She is worried about whether she will ever be able to have children. There is a lack of breast development and other secondary sexual characteristics and she is of short stature.

THEME: COLONIC DISORDERS

Options

A   Carcinoma of the caecum

B   Carcinoma of the sigmoid colon

C   Colonic polyp

D   Crohn disease

E   Diverticulitis

F   Haemorrhoids

G   Irritable bowel syndrome

H   Sigmoid volvulus

I   Ulcerative colitis

For each patient below, choose the most appropriate diagnosis from the list of options above. Each option may be used once, more than once or not at all.

☐ **13.60** A 72-year-old man presents with increasing tiredness over a 2-year period. He has microcytic anaemia and a mass in the right iliac fossa.

☐ **13.61** A 33-year-old woman consults you regarding symptoms of alternating diarrhoea and constipation associated with cramp-like abdominal pain.

☐ **13.62** A 76-year-old man presents with weight loss, pain on eating and abdominal distension. Plain abdominal X-ray films show the so-called 'coffee bean' sign.

☐ **13.63** An 82-year-old woman presents to accident and emergency with a distended abdomen. A plain abdominal X-ray film shows gross faecal loading in the colon and gas in the small bowel. The rectum is empty.

☐ **13.64** A 39-year-old woman presents with passage of bloodstained motions and mucus five times a day. Symptoms have persisted for over 1 month and are associated with weight loss. Barium enema shows no evidence of a colonic neoplasm, but a granular mucosa.

THEME: MONITORING OF DRUGS

Options

A Amiodarone

B Azathioprine

C Levodopa

D Lithium

E Phenytoin

F Ramipril

G Simvastatin

H Warfarin

For each monitoring regimen below select the single most likely drug from the list above to which it applies. Each option may be used once, more than once or not at all.

☐ **13.65** Measure blood levels after each change of dose.

☐ **13.66** Do a full blood count weekly for 4 weeks, thereafter every 3 months.

☐ **13.67** Measure serum concentrations every 3 months and thyroid function every 6 months.

☐ **13.68** Measure renal function before starting, after 1 month and yearly during treatment.

THEME: CAUSES OF A SORE MOUTH

Options

A Antibiotic associated candidosis

B Burning mouth syndrome

C Coated tongue

D Geographic tongue

E Iron deficiency

F Lichen planus

G Oral hairy leucoplakia

H Squamous cell carcinoma

I Systemic lupus erythematosus

J Thrush

K Trauma

L Vitamin B_{12} deficiency

For each of the following scenarios, choose the most likely diagnosis from the list of options above. Each option may be used once, more than once or not at all.

☐ **13.69 A 20-year-old woman has become concerned about recurrent episodes of tongue soreness exacerbated by spicy foods. She says that she has seen areas of erythematous smooth red areas on her tongue which seem to move over the weeks.**

☐ **13.70 A 65-year-old heavy smoker has had a long-standing increasingly painful ulcer on the lateral border of his tongue. He first noticed the ulcer 3 months ago and he is now having difficulty speaking.**

☐ **13.71 A 55-year-old woman with a pruritic skin rash affecting her wrists and shins has also noticed oral soreness. On examination of her mouth there are areas of white striae and ulceration affecting her tongue and buccal mucosa.**

☐ **13.72** A 70-year-old woman is found to have a smooth, sore, red tongue with soreness and cracking at the corners of her mouth. She is undergoing investigation for a mass in her right iliac fossa.

☐ **13.73** A 23-year-old man with asthma complains of a sore mouth. On examination he is found to have an inflamed palate with white specks and a smooth red tongue.

THEME: CHILD WITH A PAINFUL LEG

Options

A Fractured femur

B Irritable hip

C Non-accidental injury

D Osgood–Schlatter disease

E Osteomyelitis

F Perthes disease

G Septic arthritis

H Shin splints

I Sickle cell disease

J Slipped femoral epiphysis

For each of the patients below, choose the single most likely diagnosis from the list of options above. Each option may be used once, more than once or not at all.

☐ **13.74** A 5-year-old boy has a painful limp for a few weeks. Examination reveals limited movement at the hip. X-ray of the hip shows sclerosis of the femoral head. The parents deny any trauma.

☐ **13.75** A 13-year-old boy who is overweight develops hip pain after a minor fall. An X-ray of the hip shows abnormal findings.

☐ **13.76** A 12-year-old child who enjoys sports develops a tender tibial tuberosity.

☐ **13.77** A 6-year-old boy develops a limp after an upper respiratory tract infection. X-rays show normal findings.

☐ **13.78** A 5-month-old girl is brought in to the emergency department by her nanny because she has been crying all morning. Her left thigh is swollen. There is no history of trauma.

13.79 A 26-year-old woman developed a high fever and vomiting on the third day of her period. She then developed a macular erythematous rash over her face and trunk, associated with confusion, conjunctival suffusion, peripheral oedema and a strawberry-like appearance of her tongue.

Select the single most probable diagnosis from the list below.

- ☐ **A** Stevens–Johnson syndrome
- ☐ **B** Toxic epidermal necrolysis
- ☐ **C** Toxic shock syndrome
- ☐ **D** Typhoid fever
- ☐ **E** Yellow fever

13.80 A 21-year-old woman has several localised papular lesions on her hands and feet. One of the partners in the practice has seen her and diagnosed granuloma annulare.

Select the single most appropriate investigation for this woman from the list below.

- ☐ **A** Fasting blood sugar
- ☐ **B** HbA1c level
- ☐ **C** Skin biopsy
- ☐ **D** Skin scraping for fungal culture
- ☐ **E** Thyroid function tests

13.81 Which one of the following diseases is not notifiable under the Public Health Act 1984 and Public Health Regulations 1988?

- [ ] **A** Food poisoning
- [ ] **B** Mumps
- [ ] **C** Parvovirus infection
- [ ] **D** Scarlet fever
- [ ] **E** Whooping cough

13.82 A 52-year-old postmenopausal woman presents with general fatigue. Blood tests show that her serum aminotransferase level is 160 IU/l and alkaline phosphatase level is 185 U/l with bilirubin 35 μmol/l. A full blood count shows mild normocytic normochromic anaemia with thrombocytopenia and leucopenia. Liver biopsy shows chronic inflammatory cell infiltrate with lymphocytes, plasma cells and sometimes lymphoid follicles in the portal tracts. (Normal values: bilirubin 3–17 μmol/l, alanine aminotransferase 5–35 IU/l, alkaline phosphatase 30–150 U/l. Select the single most probable diagnosis from the list below.

- [ ] **A** α_1-AT deficiency
- [ ] **B** Autoimmune hepatitis
- [ ] **C** Chronic hepatitis C infection
- [ ] **D** Infectious mononucleosis
- [ ] **E** Non-alcoholic steatohepatitis (NASH)

CHAPTER 13 QUESTIONS

13.83 Which of the following is an indication of a severe, life-threatening asthma exacerbation?

- ☐ **A** Peak expiratory flow rate (PEFR) < 50% best or predicted
- ☐ **B** Reduced response to β$_2$-agonist inhaler
- ☐ **C** Stridor
- ☐ **D** Tachypnoea > 25 breaths/minute
- ☐ **E** Tachycardia > 100 beats/minute

13.84 A 45-year-old woman presents with neck and arm pain.

Which of the following signs if present should lead to prompt neurosurgical referral?

- ☐ **A** Brisk biceps reflex
- ☐ **B** Decreased grip strength
- ☐ **C** Decreased pronator jerk
- ☐ **D** Loss of sensation in the little finger
- ☐ **E** Neck stiffness

13.85 Which one of the following people has the greatest risk of attempting suicide?

- ☐ **A** 17-year-old student who has recently split from her boyfriend
- ☐ **B** 24-year-old unemployed single man
- ☐ **C** 34-year-old mother with postnatal depression
- ☐ **D** 62-year-old widow who has recently been diagnosed with depression
- ☐ **E** 78-year-old man with exacerbation of his chronic obstructive pulmonary disease.

13.86   Which one of the following is not a risk factor for stroke?

- ☐ **A**   Atrial fibrillation
- ☐ **B**   Diabetes mellitus
- ☐ **C**   Hypertension
- ☐ **D**   Hypothyroidism
- ☐ **E**   Obesity

13.87   A 38-year-old woman, 10 days' post partum, presents with a history of foul-smelling discharge per vagina. She has been passing blood clots per vagina for 24 hours. Her blood pressure is 90/40 mmHg, pulse 110 beats/minute, and temperature 38°C. Her uterus is tender on palpation and the fundus reaches the umbilicus.

Select the single most probable diagnosis from the list below.

- ☐ **A**   Cervical tear
- ☐ **B**   Menorrhagia
- ☐ **C**   Pelvic inflammatory disease
- ☐ **D**   Primary post-partum haemorrhage
- ☐ **E**   Secondary post-partum haemorrhage

13.88   A 56-year-old man presents with pinkish-red scaly plaques on the extensor surface of his knees and elbow. The lesions are itchy and sore.

What would be the most appropriate single first-line treatment for this condition?

- ☐ **A**   Calcipotriol
- ☐ **B**   Dithranol
- ☐ **C**   Oral steroids
- ☐ **D**   Phototherapy (UVB and UVA)
- ☐ **E**   Topical steroids

CHAPTER 13 QUESTIONS

13.89 Which one of the following drugs causes gingival hyperplasia?

- [ ] **A** Allopurinol
- [ ] **B** Atenolol
- [ ] **C** Phenytoin
- [ ] **D** Ramipril
- [ ] **E** Sodium valproate

13.90 Which one of the following statements about statins is correct?

- [ ] **A** All patients with hypertension should be taking a statin
- [ ] **B** Patients with a 10-year cardiovascular disease risk of more than 20% should receive a statin for primary prevention
- [ ] **C** Patients with type 2 diabetes should have their cardiovascular risk calculated to assess their need for a statin
- [ ] **D** Statins are better than fibrates in reducing triglyceride levels
- [ ] **E** They should only be prescribed for patients with established coronary heart disease

13.91 A 56-year-old man has recently had some blood tests performed by the practice nurse. He comes to see you, worried he may have diabetes because he has been very thirsty and has lost some weight.

Which one of the following results would confirm this diagnosis?

- [ ] **A** Fasting glucose: 6.9 mmol/l
- [ ] **B** Fasting glucose: 8.1 mmol/l
- [ ] **C** Glucose 1 hour after oral glucose tolerance test: 10.8 mmol/l
- [ ] **D** HbA1c: 8.2%
- [ ] **E** Random glucose: 9.2 mmol/l

13.92   Which one of the following is not a normal variant in babies?

☐ **A**   A 12-hour-old baby with jaundice

☐ **B**   An urticarial looking rash on a 3-day-old baby

☐ **C**   Blue looking feet in a 1-day-old baby

☐ **D**   Non-retractile foreskin in a 6-month-old boy

☐ **E**   Sneezing in a 2-hour-old baby

☐ **F**   Tiny cream pearls on the hard palate in a newborn baby

☐ **G**   Very dry skin in a newborn baby born at 42 weeks' gestation

13.93   A 30-year-old mountain biker who frequently competes on forest terrain complains of a flu-like illness, splenomegaly and arthralgia.

Select the single most likely cause from the list below.

☐ **A**   *Borrelia burgdorferi* infection

☐ **B**   Fasciolopsiasis

☐ **C**   Filariasis

☐ **D**   Giardiasis

☐ **E**   Toxacariasis

CHAPTER 13 QUESTIONS

13.94 A 67-year-old woman who consumes a low-fibre diet presents with a short history of lower abdominal pain, more so in the left iliac fossa (LIF), associated with nausea and constipation. She can tolerate oral fluids. On examination you note she looks mildly unwell with a temperature of 37.5°C.

Select from the list below the next most appropriate step in management.

- ☐ **A** Admit urgently to surgical team for assessment
- ☐ **B** Arrange a barium enema X-ray
- ☐ **C** Increase her laxatives and review in 1 week
- ☐ **D** Prescribe an anti-spasmodic drug
- ☐ **E** Treat with broad-spectrum antibiotics

13.95 A 68-year-old woman presents to her GP with general symptoms of tiredness, weight loss and sweating during the night. She seems to be generally depressed. Further enquiry reveals she has stiffness and pain in her shoulders and neck, which is worse in the morning and lasts about 30 minutes.

What is the single best investigation for this condition from the list below?

- ☐ **A** Autoantibody screen
- ☐ **B** Erythrocyte sedimentation rate (ESR)
- ☐ **C** Muscle biopsy
- ☐ **D** Nerve conduction velocity
- ☐ **E** Temporal artery biopsy

13.96 A 32-year-old man diagnosed as having type 1 diabetes mellitus was started on Mixtard insulin. However, control proved to be a problem, with hypoglycaemia between meals and particularly at night. This was substituted with rapid-acting insulin analogues, but has resulted in erratic morning blood sugar readings.

Which one of the following is the single best management option to overcome this problem?

- [ ] **A** Add a sulphonylurea
- [ ] **B** Add insulin glargine
- [ ] **C** Add the new class of insulin secretagogues – repaglinide
- [ ] **D** Add twice daily medium-acting insulin
- [ ] **E** Adjust the dose of a rapid-acting insulin according to blood glucose results

13.97 A 62-year-old politician has been finding it increasingly difficult to remember all the information at his daily party meetings. This has been followed by a decline in language function: he finds it difficult to remember the names of his colleagues, and planning, organising and abstracting have also become difficult. Now, at times, he also becomes agitated and aggressive. There is a history of similar deterioration of function in the family.

Select the single most likely diagnosis from the list below.

- [ ] **A** Alzheimer disease
- [ ] **B** Creutzfeldt–Jakob disease
- [ ] **C** Lewy body dementia
- [ ] **D** Multi-infarct dementia
- [ ] **E** Parkinson disease

13.98 A 20-week pregnant woman has a recent history of indirect exposure to chickenpox as one of her neighbour's children has chickenpox. The patient is not sure whether she had chickenpox as a child.

Select the single best management for this patient from the list below.

- [ ] **A** Aciclovir
- [ ] **B** Check for serum varicella zoster IgG
- [ ] **C** Immunoglobulins and aciclovir
- [ ] **D** Termination of pregnancy
- [ ] **E** Varicella zoster vaccination

13.99 Which one of the following is not a cause of reduced fertility in men?

- [ ] **A** Past history of testicular torsion
- [ ] **B** Peyronie disease
- [ ] **C** Previous mumps infection
- [ ] **D** Smoking
- [ ] **E** Undescended testicle

13.100 A 24-year-old man presents with right earache and deafness that has worsened over 24 hours. His ear has started discharging and the pain has improved.

Select the single most likely diagnosis from the list below.

- [ ] **A** Acute otitis externa
- [ ] **B** Acute otitis media
- [ ] **C** Chronic suppurative otitis media
- [ ] **D** Glue ear
- [ ] **E** Wax

ANSWERS

THEME: HYPERTENSION TREATMENT

13.1   **A**   **Amlodipine**

All patients with diabetes and hypertension should be taking an ACE inhibitor, unless it is contraindicated. β-Blockers should not be used to treat hypertension in diabetic patients (unless they are needed for coronary heart disease). Diuretics are sometimes used for diabetic patients but would not be used first or even second line. (www.nice.org.uk/Cg34).

13.2   **E**   **Lisinopril**

The National Institute for Health and Clinical Excellence (NICE) guidelines state that calicum channel blockers or thiazide diuretics should be used first line for black patients at any age. An ACE inhibitor should be added to the initial therapy if the blood pressure is not controlled.

13.3   **B**   **Atenolol**

β-blockers are still used for coronary heart disease and would be very suitable for this patient. β-blockers are no longer used as first line treatment as studies have shown that they are less effective at reducing cardiovascular events.

13.4   **F**   **Losartan**

Angiotensin-II receptor blockers would be suitable for this woman as it appears she has developed an ACE-related cough. She should be reviewed to ensure her cough improves on stopping the ACE inhibitor. Around 10% of patients taking ACE inhibitors develop an ACE inhibitor cough.

13.5 G Methyl dopa

Sustained hypertension greater than 160/100 mmHg in pregnancy is usually an indication for treatment. Hypertension increases the risk of pre-eclampsia and placental abruption. The centrally acting agent methyl dopa is the drug of choice. Labetalol, nifedipine and hydralazine are also sometimes used.

THEME: INFECTIOUS DISEASES IN CHILDHOOD

13.6 E Symptomatic relief (antipyretics and/or analgesics)

This is likely to be infectious mononucleosis, most commonly caused by the Epstein–Barr virus. It typically infects older children and is spread via oral secretions. Other features include tonsillitis/pharyngitis, splenomegaly, hepatomegaly, jaundice, maculopapular rash. Symptoms may persist for some months but treatment is symptomatic.

13.7 E Symptomatic relief (antipyretics and/or analgesics)

This is most likely varicella zoster infection (chickenpox). Spread is by the respiratory route and it has a 14-day incubation period. Most patients will become symptomatic with the infection. It is highly infectious. Crops of new spots occur for typically 3–5 days then the lesions crust over. Uncomplicated infection in a child who is not immunocompromised requires only symptomatic treatment.

13.8 B Intravenous antibiotic

This is scalded skin syndrome – a staphylococcal skin infection. Typically the skin is red and tender and areas of epidermis may separate on gentle pressure (Nikolsky sign). Intravenous antibiotics are required as this is a serious infection.

13.9   C   Oral aciclovir

This is primary herpes simplex infection. The *British National Formulary* recommends a soft diet, adequate fluid, analgesia and the use of chlorhexidine mouthwash. In the case of severe herpes stomatitis, systemic aciclovir is required. There is no suggestion that this child is immunocompromised so the oral route seems appropriate.

13.10   G   Topical antibiotic

This is likely to be conjunctivitis. The conjunctiva will be red and inflamed. It can be allergic, bacterial or viral in nature. The presence of a purulent discharge, however, suggests a bacterial origin, and topical antibiotic drops or ointment will be appropriate.

THEME: CHEST PAIN

13.11   C   Chest infection

It is very likely that this woman has a chest infection. She is more prone to chest infections as she has chronic obstructive pulmonary disease. She has some pleuritic chest pain which is classically worse on deep inspiration. She should be treated with antibiotics and anti-inflammatory analgesics.

13.12   G   Pulmonary embolism

Pulmonary embolism is the most likely diagnosis for this woman. There is an increased risk of venous thromboembolism post partum. Her legs should be examined for any clinical signs of deep vein thrombosis and she should be admitted to hospital.

13.13   D   Musculoskeletal pain

This is the most likely diagnosis as the history is not typical for angina. However, it is important to exclude angina as being a smoker, he is at an increased risk of coronary heart disease. His risk factors for coronary heart disease should be addressed in this consultation.

13.14   I   Unstable angina

This woman has unstable angina as it is occurring at rest. She is at a high risk of having another myocardial infarction and should be admitted to hospital.

13.15   F   Oesophageal reflux

It is most likely that the anti-inflammatory drug he is taking for his wrist has caused some gastric irritation leading to indigestion and reflux symptoms. He should stop taking ibuprofen.

THEME: FACIAL RASHES

13.16   A   Acne vulgaris

Acne is very common – affecting around 50% of teenagers with varying severity. Despite various beliefs, acne is not usually worsened by eating chocolate. Acne usually worsens during puberty.

13.17   B   Actinic keratoses

Actinic keratoses are due to prolonged and repeated solar exposure and hence are more common on the face and scalp. The scale is quite adherent and only removed with difficulty and pain. The skin is rough like sandpaper. Highly hypertrophic lesions and cutaneous horns may require biopsy to exclude squamous cell carcinoma.

13.18   D   Perioral dermatitis

This is most likely to be perioral dermatitis. Topical steroids exacerbate the condition. Treatment is with topical or systemic antibiotics.

13.19   F   Rosacea

Rosacea is the most likely diagnosis. It can often be confused with acne vulgaris in which there are comedones, a wider distribution and improvement with sunlight. Topical steroids should be avoided in patients with rosacea because they exacerbate the condition. Sunlight and alcohol also can make it worse.

13.20   G   Seborrhoeic eczema

Skin infection by yeast called *Pityrosporum* is thought to play a part in seborrhoeic eczema. Anti-yeast treatment can therefore be effective, although it usually needs to be repeated periodically. A mixture of antifungal cream and mild steroid (1% hydrocortisone) is the usual regimen for flare-ups.

THEME: MACROSCOPIC HAEMATURIA

13.21   F   Renal cancer

As the woman cannot see the colour of her urine she may have had haematuria for a long time. Broken bones after trivial injury raise the possibility of pathological fracture and renal cancer typically metastasises to bone (and lungs).

13.22　J　Ureteric calculus

Stones affect men more than women and one of the classic sites where ureteric stones get lodged is the vesicoureteric junction (VUJ). Here irritation of the trigone leads to frequency and as the detrusor muscle squeezes down on itself to empty the bladder it also squeezes the stone in the VUJ leading to pain at the end of micturition.

13.23　H　Schistosomiasis

Schistosomiasis is endemic in Egypt ('the land of menstruating men,' Herodotus) and bacterial cystitis typically coexists with the bilharzial infection, exacerbating the situation.

13.24　A　Bladder cancer

Even if the international normalised ratio (INR) is too high, bleeding usually occurs if there is an abnormality somewhere along the urinary tract, and therefore patients taking warfarin need to be investigated as thoroughly as other patients. This patient is an elderly person with frank painless haematuria and therefore has approximately a 25% chance of harbouring a bladder cancer.

13.25　C　Haemorrhagic cystitis

Urinary infection is a potent cause of confusion in elderly people, and one needs to be concerned why she is not improving with the antibiotics. Either it is an unusual organism or there is a predisposing factor such as a large post-void residual making elimination of infected urine inefficient (and contributing to long-standing urinary incontinence). Once the bladder urothelium is severely and chronically inflamed it will start to bleed.

THEME: SHORT STATURE IN CHILDREN

13.26   A   Achondroplasia

Disproportionately shortened limbs would point to a skeletal dysplasia such as achondroplasia. This is an autosomal dominant condition.

13.27   F   Noonan syndrome

Noonan syndrome in boys mimics many of the features of Turner syndrome. However, Turner occurs only in girls as it is due to the chromosomal defect XO.

13.28   D   Growth hormone deficiency

Cranial irradiation especially at a young age can lead to hypopituitarism and loss of growth hormone production, further resulting in short stature and hypoglycaemia.

13.29   B   Congenital hypothyroidism

The child has congenital hypothyroidism. It is usually detected by neonatal screening before the signs are evident.

THEME: CAUSES OF A NON-BLANCHING RASH

13.30   E   Henoch–Schönlein purpura

Henoch–Schönlein purpura is a hypersensitivity reaction, sometimes preceded by an upper respiratory tract infection. Associated problems include arthralgia, abdominal pain and microscopic haematuria. Glomerulonephritis can progress to renal failure. The main treatment is with analgesics.

13.31   F   Immune thrombocytopenic purpura

This is an immune disorder characterised by platelet-bound antibodies. There is often a previous history of infection. Most episodes resolve over a few months but there is a danger of serious bleeding.

13.32   H   Non-accidental injury

Always consider child abuse if purpura is seen in an unusual place or shows an unusual distribution.

13.33   G   Meningococcal septicaemia

Meningococcal purpura implies significant septicaemia. Rapid deterioration is likely. Aggressive management with antibiotics, intravenous fluids, intubation and ventilation is required.

13.34   A   Acute leukaemia

The history suggests low haemoglobin and platelets as well as poor immunity. In leukaemia all three blood cell types are affected.

THEME: INVESTIGATIONS OF PRURITUS VULVAE

13.35   C   High vaginal swab

13.36   E   None of the above

13.37   A   Creatinine clearance

13.38   D   Vulval biopsy

13.39   B   Glucose tolerance test

In most cases of pruritus vulvae there is an underlying gynaecological cause. However, in a proportion of cases systemic disorders are aetiological factors such as diabetes mellitus or dermatological conditions. Poor hygiene, use of talcum powders, deodorants, bath salts, synthetic underwear, tight jeans and biological washing powders contribute to the symptoms and these should be elicited from the history. In older women with a localised lesion, a biopsy is essential.

THEME: CAUSES OF CLUBBING

13.40   J   Infective endocarditis

Infective endocarditis is easily overlooked as a cause of subacute or chronic illness in older people. However, fever and murmurs often coexist without endocarditis. Endocarditis on a previously normal valve is more common after surgical instrumentation of the urogenital or gastro-intestinal tract or after dental work. Clinical signs include clubbing, splinter haemorrhages, haematuria, retinal Roth spots (basically cotton wool spots due to vasculitis), Janeway lesions (palmar/plantar infarcted papules) and Osler nodes (painful infarcted papules on the finger pulps).

13.41   B   Bronchiectasis

Any chronic suppurative lung disease can cause clubbing. In a young or middle-aged person, the most likely diagnosis is bronchiectasis. This may be idiopathic or follow previous infection (whooping cough, tuberculosis) or bronchial obstruction, which causes localised bronchiectasis. Signs are due to fixed narrowing of some airways with excess sputum production. In a younger patient, cystic fibrosis gives a similar clinical picture, including clubbing.

CHAPTER 13 ANSWERS

13.42   E   Squamous cell lung cancer

Smoking and asbestos exposure together massively increase the risk of lung malignancy. Squamous cell carcinoma is more common than mesothelioma and Horner syndrome is usually due to an apical squamous cell cancer.

13.43   C   Coeliac disease

Cystic fibrosis, coeliac disease and Crohn disease can all cause malabsorption, growth delay and clubbing. Of these, coeliac disease is the most common condition to present at this age. Cystic fibrosis is almost always identified in young children and most will have respiratory problems at the time of diagnosis. Children with coeliac disease are often pale skinned with fair hair. Arthralgia and dermatitis herpetiformis may also occur.

13.44   A   Axillary artery aneurysm

Unilateral clubbing is rare. One cause is an axillary artery aneurysm, which is usually acquired in adulthood after trauma such as angiography via the brachial artery. Another possibility is coarctation of the aorta proximal to the origin of the right subclavian artery.

THEME: COMMON PRESENTATIONS OF SPORTSMEN/WOMEN

13.45   J   Ulnar collateral ligament rupture

This is rupture of the ulnar collateral ligament of the thumb and is a common skiing injury. The lesion is detected on stress testing. Referral for surgical repair may be necessary, especially if the proximal end of the tendon has become trapped inside the aponeurosis of the thumb adductor causing impaired abduction/adduction of the thumb. The common term is gamekeeper's thumb as it can occur when wringing a pheasant's neck!

13.46   H   Shin splints

Shin splints is pain in the anterior shin caused by either a stress fracture of the tibia, inflammation of the muscles on the anterior compartment of the lower leg or periostitis of the tibia. It is an overuse syndrome caused by poor running technique where the foot is forcibly plantarflexed against resistance from tibialis anterior. The most important diagnosis to exclude is chronic compartment syndrome, where there is so much swelling that the pressure causes muscle ischaemia, more swelling and a vicious circle. In the short term, the condition can be managed by rest, and in the long term, by improving running technique with appropriate advice from an experienced physiotherapist.

13.47   D   Lateral epicondylitis

Lateral epicondylitis is usually called tennis elbow but is also very common in other repeated activities involving forced pronation and extension of the wrist. Violinists present with right arm symptoms. Gripping and wrist extension are painful. The diagnosis is made by demonstrating tenderness over the lateral epicondyle, pain on resisted wrist extension. An important differential is cervical root pain, which is also common in violinists. Treatment is initially rest, ice and non-steroidal anti-inflammatory drugs (NSAIDs), followed by advice on technique, stretching and strengthening exercises from a specialist physiotherapist. Short term relief may be obtained by local steroid injection but this does not remove the cause so there is risk of recurrence.

13.48   B   Bucket handle meniscus tear

A bucket handle tear describes a common injury to the medial meniscus, caused by twisting with the knee flexed. The knee may lock or give way as the loose meniscus fragment lodges between the femoral condyles. The medial joint line will be tender and McMurray's test may be positive. There may be an effusion. Large tears may need removal of the loose body during arthroscopy; small tears may need no treatment. Refer for arthroscopy if symptoms are severe and interfere with functioning of the knee.

CHAPTER 13 ANSWERS

13.49   A   Anterior knee pain

Anterior knee pain (patellofemoral syndrome) is caused by irritation of the undersurface of the patella which may cause damage to the cartilage. The patella normally slides up and down the patellar groove on the anterior distal femur. If it is malaligned there is increased force of friction. Malalignment is usually caused by imbalance of forces between medial and lateral quadriceps groups, pulling the patella laterally. It is common in rowers because of the positioning, and in females because of the greater angle between tibia and femur caused by the wider pelvis. Initial treatment is rest, followed by exercises to strengthen the medial quadriceps and advice on technique.

THEME: HEADACHE

13.50   C   Migraine

Migraine is the most likely diagnosis. The patient is describing some classic features of migraine with some aura. The oral contraceptive should be stopped in view of this diagnosis. If simple analgesics are not beneficial then a triptan may be helpful.

13.51   B   Cluster headache

Cluster headaches more commonly affect men and can start at any age. They are unilateral and always on the same side. They last 20–60 minutes and may recur several times every day for several weeks. Treatment is often very difficult as analgesics do not usually relieve the pain as they take too long to work. Inhalation of 100% oxygen often relieves cluster headache for some people, particularly frequent cluster headaches that occur at night.

13.52   D   Subarachnoid haemorrhage

New headaches that start very suddenly (sometimes described like a sudden blow to the head) must be taken very seriously. Any patient who describes a very severe, sudden-onset headache needs to be admitted to hospital and investigated for a subarachnoid haemorrhage.

13.53   G   Trigeminal neuralgia

This is classic trigeminal neuralgia. The majority of cases are unilateral, in the distribution of one or more divisions of the trigeminal nerve, and occur in mid to late life. Patients often describe the pain like an electric shock, which is often precipitated by cold wind, washing the face, shaving or eating. Oral carbamazepine is usually used as first line treatment. Occasionally surgery is needed.

13.54   F   Tension headache

The pain of tension headache is typically present all day, worse in the evening. In contrast, the pain from raised intracranial pressure tends to be present on waking and persists less during the day than a tension headache. Any stresses in the patient's life should be reduced, if possible.

13.55   E   Temporal arteritis

Temporal arteritis should be diagnosed here as he has very typical symptoms. It is important not to miss this diagnosis at it is potentially sight-threatening if left untreated. High-dose steroids need to be started as soon as the diagnosis is suspected, even before a temporal artery biopsy.

CHAPTER 13 ANSWERS

THEME: FAILURE TO CONCEIVE

13.56   A   Endocervical and high vaginal swab

The history and examination findings suggest possible pelvic inflammatory disease. First line investigation would be endocervical and high vaginal swabs to detect and treat any current genital infection. Later, a hysterosalpingogram may be indicated to look for any tubal scarring but this would not be first line.

13.57   D   Pelvic ultrasound scan

This history is suggestive of polycystic ovarian syndrome (PCOS) which a normal LH/FSH ratio does not exclude. The next investigation would therefore be a pelvic ultrasound to look for the presence of polycystic ovaries. PCOS is defined as polycystic ovaries plus one or more of: amenorrhoea/oligomenorrhoea, male pattern baldness, hirsutism, acne, raised serum testosterone/LH. Management of infertility may include weight loss and treatment with metformin and clomifene.

13.58   E   Serum LH and FSH

This woman may be perimenopausal and it is important to diagnose this before embarking on other investigations. Raised LH/FSH together with low oestradiol would suggest this.

13.59   C   Karyotype analysis

This girl has features suggestive of Turner syndrome with failure of development of any secondary sexual characteristics and primary amenorrhoea. Other clinical features of Turner syndrome are shield chest, cubitus valgus, lymphoedema, short fourth metacarpal, low-set ears and hypertension. The karyotype in Turner syndrome is 45 XO.

THEME: COLONIC DISORDERS

13.60   A   Carcinoma of the caecum

Carcinoma of the caecum often presents in an insidious way, with a microcytic anaemia, weight loss and sometimes an ache or palpable mass in the right iliac fossa. The large calibre of the caecum and liquid consistency of the stool at this point allows these tumours to grow for a long period of time. Unfortunately, some of these patients receive several courses of iron tablets before the true diagnosis is made.

13.61   G   Irritable bowel syndrome

Irritable bowel syndrome is a diagnosis of exclusion, which typically occurs in younger patients and may be associated with stress or dietary intolerance. Symptoms include constipation or diarrhoea or both together, along with cramp-like abdominal pains. Treatment with anti-spasmodic agents, fibre, or exclusion diets can be tried, although any organic pathology must be ruled out at first.

13.62   H   Sigmoid volvulus

Sigmoid volvulus is more common in equatorial countries where the diet is rich in fibre. However, it does occur in temperate countries and usually presents with symptoms of pain and bloating, sometimes as an emergency. A plain abdominal film may demonstrate a large double colonic loop, which is said to resemble a coffee bean.

CHAPTER 13 ANSWERS

13.63   B   Carcinoma of the sigmoid colon

Left-sided colonic tumours will more commonly present with an obstructive picture than right-sided tumours. This is due to the more narrow calibre of the colon combined with the more solid consistency of its contents at this point. Typically an annular constricting carcinoma will present with an alteration in bowel habit, change in stool calibre, and finally, frank obstruction. A plain abdominal film may show gross faecal loading proximal to this point, with an absence of bowel gas distally. A contrast enema will usually confirm the diagnosis.

13.64   I   Ulcerative colitis

Ulcerative colitis is a disease of unknown aetiology which tends to affect people in the third and fourth decade of life (15% are under the age of 15). It usually presents as a chronic relatively low-grade illness, although 15% of patients may present with fulminant disease. Symptoms include blood-stained diarrhoea, abdominal pain and fever. Extracolonic manifestations include arthritis, iritis, hepatic dysfunction and cutaneous manifestations. The ulceration is superficial, unlike the transmural disease seen in Crohn colitis.

THEME: MONITORING OF DRUGS

13.65   E   Phenytoin

The relationship between dose and plasma concentration is not linear. Small dose increases may produce large increases in plasma concentrations with a risk of toxic effects.

13.66   B   Azathioprine

There is a risk of bone marrow depression.

13.67   D   Lithium

Lithium salts have a narrow therapeutic/toxic ratio. Doses are adjusted to achieve a serum concentration of 0.4–1.0 mmol/l on samples taken 12 hours after a dose. Lithium also causes hypothyroidism.

13.68   F   Ramipril

Angiotensin-converting enzyme (ACE) inhibitors are likely to cause progressive renal failure in patients with renal artery stenosis and in certain other situations.

THEME: CAUSES OF A SORE MOUTH

13.69   D   Geographic tongue

Geographic tongue or erythema migrans is a common autosomal dominant inherited condition that may affect up to 5% of the population. The dorsum of the tongue is affected with migratory areas of depapillation, which may be surrounded by whitish margins. It is often asymptomatic but may give rise to concern when first noticed by the patient or if it leads to soreness while eating spicy food.

13.70   H   Squamous cell carcinoma

Oral squamous cell carcinoma is the commonest oral malignancy. Its preferred site is the U-shaped area in the floor of the mouth that lies between and includes the lateral border of the tongue and the mucosa covering the lingual aspect of mandibular alveolar bone. Note that a biopsy should be done for any oral ulcer which has persisted for more than 2 weeks to exclude malignancy. White and red patches in the mouth may be dysplastic or represent carcinoma.

13.71   F   Lichen planus

Lichen planus is a mucocutaneous disorder of possibly immunological aetiology. The eruption both on the skin and in the mouth tends to be symmetrical. On the skin it tends to start on the flexor surfaces with red and then violaceous pruritic, polygonal, papules which may have white 'Wickham' striae on their surface. In about 50% of patients the skin lesions resolve within 9 months. Oral lesions tend to continue for much longer and may be reticular, atrophic or ulcerative. The genitalia may also be involved. Lichen planus, like psoriasis, viral warts and vitiligo, shows the Koebner phenomenon.

13.72   E   Iron deficiency

Iron deficiency may present initially with angular cheilitis and a smooth, red, depapillated, sore tongue. The cause of iron deficiency in this patient may be an occult caecal carcinoma.

13.73   J   Thrush

Poor steroid inhaler technique often results in patients with asthma developing steroid-associated oral candidosis or thrush which may cause an erythematous appearance of the dorsum of the tongue and opposing palate. All patients starting to use such inhalers should have their technique checked, should rinse their mouth after inhaler use and if possible use a spacer device to increase delivery of the corticosteroid to the lungs.

THEME: CHILD WITH A PAINFUL LEG

13.74   F   Perthes disease

Perthes disease generally presents with limp, with or without pain, between the ages of 4 and 8 years. Avascular necrosis of the femoral head occurs followed by replacement with new bone. The patient can be left with residual femoral head deformity. Other causes of avascular necrosis in children are sickle cell disease and prolonged steroid use. It unlikely to be sickle cell disease as this would be associated with severe pain and there would have been a history of other crises by the age of 5 years.

13.75   J   Slipped femoral epiphysis

Slipped upper femoral epiphysis can present with pain and a limp of gradual onset, or more acutely after minor trauma. It presents at this age and classically in obese boys with delayed secondary sexual development.

13.76   D   Osgood–Schlatter disease

This is a traction apophysitis at the insertion of the patella tendon into the tibial tubercle. Tenderness over the tubercle and changes seen on X-ray confirm the diagnosis. Treatment involves reducing the strain at this site by stopping sports or by immobilisation.

13.77   B   Irritable hip

In this age group the joint may become inflamed after an upper respiratory tract infection. The exact cause is not known but it causes an irritable hip or transient synovitis. Blood tests and X-rays show normal findings. Most cases resolve in a few days or weeks. This diagnosis is only made once all investigations are demonstrated to be normal.

13.78 C Non-accidental injury

The pathological diagnosis is likely to be fractured femur. However, the clinical diagnosis may be non-accidental injury. Infants are unlikely to break their bones without some external force. Children may be brought in by carers other than the parents. A senior paediatric opinion must be sought immediately while you attend to the child's injury.

13.79 C Toxic shock syndrome

Toxic shock syndrome usually occurs in the setting of staphylococcal infection of skin or soft tissues, and is mediated by the endotoxin TSS-1. Characteristic clinical features also include hypotension, shock and very high body temperatures (> 39.5°C). Treatment is predominantly with supportive care to ensure adequate circulating volume, administration of pressor agents to maintain systemic blood pressure and antibiotic treatment. The first thing to do is to remove the tampon, which is the likely source of the infection in this case.

13.80 A Fasting blood sugar

Granuloma annulare is seen more commonly in women, especially under 30 years. It is associated with type 1 diabetes, which can be diagnosed by fasting glucose. HbA1c is not sensitive enough to test for diabetes. It is harmless and self-limiting.

13.81   C   Parvovirus infection

Parvovirus causes erythema infectiosum (Fifth disease) characterised by a prodromal illness with fever followed by an erythematous facial rash (slapped cheek appearance).

The following diseases are notifiable: acute encephalitis; acute poliomyelitis; anthrax; cholera; diphtheria; dysentery; food poisoning; leptospirosis; malaria; measles; meningitis (meningococcal, pneumococcal, *Haemophilus influenzae*, viral, other specified, unspecified); meningococcal septicaemia (without meningitis); mumps; ophthalmia neonatorum; paratyphoid fever; plague; rabies; relapsing fever; rubella; scarlet fever; smallpox; tetanus; tuberculosis; typhoid fever; typhus fever; viral haemorrhagic fever; viral hepatitis (hepatitis A, hepatitis B, hepatitis C, other); whooping cough; yellow fever; and leprosy.

13.82   B   Autoimmune hepatitis

There are two peaks according to age in the presentation. Patients in the perimenopausal age group present with non-specific symptoms, whereas adolescents and people in their early twenties present with acute hepatitis and with jaundice and higher aminotransferase levels, which do not improve with time. Three types of autoimmune hepatitis have been recognised:

- type I with antibodies (antinuclear anti-smooth muscle)

- type II with antibodies (anti-LKM1)

- type III with soluble liver antigen.

Type II mostly occurs in girls and young women.

13.83   D   Tachypnoea > 25 breaths/minute

PEFR in an acute severe attack is less than 33% predicted, and tachycardia is over 120 beats/minute. Other signs of life-threatening asthma include use of accessory muscles, inability to complete sentences in one breath, confusion or exhaustion and silent chest. Acute attacks may build up over minute, hours or days, and there may be a wide range of precipitants. These include smoking, infection, stress, allergens, exercise and neglect of medications.

13.84   A   Brisk biceps reflex

Brisk reflexes are an upper motor neurone sign and suggest spinal cord compression above the level of lesion. There may be lower motor neurone signs at the level of the lesion. The level of biceps reflex is C5–6. The other signs are all common in self-limiting cervicalgia.

13.85   B   24-year-old unemployed single man

Although all of the above people do have an increased risk of attempting suicide, the risk is greatest in the young man. Single, unemployed men from the lower social classes have a high risk of suicide, and any voiced intention must be taken very seriously in the consultation.

13.86   D   Hypothyroidism

All the other options are established risk factors for stroke. Primary prevention of stroke is very important in primary care. Much of the responsibility for delivering effective secondary prevention and managing longer-term problems associated with stroke now falls to the primary care team.

13.87   E   Secondary post-partum haemorrhage

The difference between primary and secondary post-partum haemorrhage (PPH) is the timing of bleeding after delivery. Primary PPH usually occurs 24–48 hours after delivery, whereas secondary PPH can occur from 48 hours up to 14 days after delivery. In this clinical scenario, secondary PPH is due to endometritis (an infection caused by bacterial penetration of the residual stratum basalis of the endometrium), as suggested by the raised temperature, offensive vaginal discharge and tender uterus. The underlying aggravating factor may be retained products of conception, which provide a rich culture medium for the growth of bacteria.

13.88   A   Calcipotriol

The diagnosis here is psoriasis. Topical calcipotriol is better accepted by patients then dithranol and shows good evidence for inducing remission. It is easier to apply to multiple lesions and causes less skin irritation. For very inflamed lesions this can be combined with topical steroid therapy. Lesions unresponsive to topical therapy may respond to phototherapy (UVB and UVA) or systemic therapy (methotrexate, acitretin, ciclosporin or hydroxyurea).

13.89   C   Phenytoin

Gingival overgrowth, also known as gingival hyperplasia secondary to drugs, was first reported in the literature in the early 1960s in institutionalised epileptic children receiving phenytoin for the treatment of seizures. Ciclosporin and calcium channel blockers (especially nifedipine) have also been associated with gingival overgrowth. In patients taking phenytoin it is more likely to occur in the presence of gingivitis and dental plaque. Increased dental plaque induces local inflammation and may serve as a reservoir for the drug.

CHAPTER 13 ANSWERS

13.90   B   Patients with a 10-year cardiovascular disease risk of more than 20% should receive a statin for primary prevention

Statins are now widely prescribed for both primary and secondary prevention of coronary heart disease (CHD). All type 2 diabetic patients should be receiving a statin for primary prevention of cardiovascular disease (unless contraindicated). Fibrates are used first line to lower very high triglyceride levels. Only hypertensive patients with a 10-year risk of more than 20% should be considered for a statin.

13.91   B   Fasting glucose 8.1 mmol/l

The World Health Organization's publication *Definition, Diagnosis and Classification of Diabetes Mellitus and its Complications* (1999) defines the diagnostic criteria as follows:

Diabetes symptoms (ie polyuria, polydipsia and unexplained weight loss) plus

- a random venous plasma glucose concentration ≥ 11.1 mmol/l

or

- a fasting plasma glucose concentration ≥ 7.0 mmol/l (whole blood ≥ 6.1mmol/l)

or

- 2-hour plasma glucose concentration ≥ 11.1 mmol/l 2 hours after 75 g anhydrous glucose in an oral glucose tolerance test (OGTT).

When there are no symptoms, diagnosis should not be based on a single glucose determination and requires confirmatory plasma venous determination. At least one additional glucose test result on another day with a value in the diabetic range is essential: fasting, from a random sample or from the 2-hour post glucose load. If the fasting or random values are not diagnostic the 2-hour value should be used. HbA1c should never be used to diagnose diabetes.

13.92   A   A 12-hour-old baby with jaundice

Jaundice that appears in less than 24 hours may be pathological and needs to be investigated. All other answers are normal variants in babies. The rash described in F refers to Epstein's pearls and in B refers to erythema toxicum (neonatal urticaria) which are both normal. A newborn baby commonly sneezes to remove amniotic fluid from the nose. Blue hands and feet are common in the first few days of life in a baby. Post-dates babies often have very dry skin.

13.93   A   *Borrelia burgdorferi* infection

Borrelia causes Lyme disease, treated with doxycycline or erythromycin. Strictly speaking it is a spirochaete, but the deer tick which transmits it is a parasite. In the UK it is endemic in Thetford, Norfolk, and the New Forest, the Lake District, the Scottish Highlands and the uplands of Wales. Twenty per cent of patients with Lyme disease do not remember any tick bites and do not complain of a rash. If the tick bites at the nymph stage it is often not felt due to local anaesthetic secretions. The initial rash known as erythema chronicum migrans is a macule or papule at the bite site that expands to form an annular lesion with a distinct red border and a partially clearing centre.

13.94   E   Treat with broad-spectrum antibiotics

This scenario describes a patient with diverticulitis. Features on history are the lower abdominal pain/LIF pain with nausea and constipation. The patient may look flushed. It is more common with age, and in females. A low fibre diet is a risk factor. As this woman is able to tolerate fluids and you do not suspect any complications such as obstruction or abscess, then appropriate management is with broad-spectrum antibiotics, such as ciprofloxacin and metronidazole, for one week and a clear liquid diet.

13.95   B   ESR

Polymyalgia rheumatica is characterised by raised ESR and C-reactive protein (CRP) levels. The diagnosis should be questioned if these levels are not raised. Serum alkaline phosphatase and γ-glutamyl transferase may also be elevated. A temporal artery biopsy shows giant-cell arteritis in about 10–30% of cases, but is usually not done.

13.96   B   Add insulin glargine

Insulin glargine has reduced solubility due to its modified structure, thus prolonging its duration of action. Therefore it has a less peaked concentration profile in the blood than conventional long-acting insulins. NICE guidelines (www.formulary.cht.nhs.uk/Guidelines/NICE/053_Insulin_Glargine.htm) recommend that it should be available for those whose lifestyle is considerably restricted by recurrent symptomatic hypoglycaemia.

13.97   A   Alzheimer disease

People particularly at risk of developing Alzheimer disease are those with a family history of the disease, those who have sustained a head injury or those who have Down syndrome. Neuropathological changes include neuronal reduction, neurofibrillary tangles, senile neurotic plaques and a variable amyloid angiopathy. Aggregation of amyloid appears to be a central event. The gene for the amyloid precursor protein (APP) is localised close to the defect on chromosome 21. Dementia is diagnosed clinically from the patient's history and examination, especially cognitive testing, and it can be confirmed by psychometric testing.

13.98   B   Check for serum varicella zoster IgG

If a susceptible mother is exposed to a source of varicella zoster virus, then this may result in primary varicella infection in pregnancy. Maternal varicella in the first 20 weeks of pregnancy carries a 1–2% risk of varicella embryopathy syndrome developing in the fetus. The consequences of fetal varicella syndrome include scarring of the skin, hypoplasia of limbs and chorioretinitis. Adult varicella can cause pneumonitis as a serious complication. In the absence of symptoms, positive IgG antibody levels is highly suggestive of past infection and hence immunity.

13.99   E   Peyronie disease

Peyronie disease presents with hard lumps in the shaft of the penis and pain and bending on erection. The cause is unknown. Although it can cause erectile dysfunction, it does not affect fertility or sperm count. All of the other answers are well recognised causes of reduced fertility in men.

3.100   B   Acute otitis media

The history is short so this is an acute condition. In otitis externa the pain would not improve when the ear discharges. In otitis media a rupture of the tympanic membrane releasing discharge reduces the pain. Glue ear and wax usually just produce deafness.

CHAPTER 13 ANSWERS

Professional Dilemmas

INTRODUCTION TO PROFESSIONAL DILEMMA QUESTIONS

Professional dilemma questions make up the second 90-minute paper in the Stage 2 assessment process of appointment to general practitioner (GP) specialty training. The paper focuses on a candidate's approach to practising medicine. It consists of scenarios encapsulating a professional dilemma that might be met when practising as a doctor. Candidates have to answer how to deal with them. Thus the paper is designed to assess understanding of appropriate behaviour for a doctor in difficult situations and allows the demonstration of competencies such as coping with pressure, empathy and sensitivity, and professional integrity. These are three of the competencies in the national person specification for entry at ST1 level into GP training[4].

The paper does not require any specific knowledge of general practice but does assume a general familiarity with typical primary and secondary care procedures. A candidate's responses should represent appropriate behaviour for a second year foundation doctor.

The competencies that are assessed are:

- Empathy and sensitivity: This is the capacity and motivation to take into account others' perspectives and understand their concerns but without over-sensitive involvement. The patient will be treated with understanding using a non-judgemental approach and with appropriate words and actions.

- Coping with pressure: This is the ability to recognise one's own limitations and to seek help where necessary. It requires coping mechanisms to remain under control of difficult situations, maintain the wider focus and respond appropriately when faced with the unexpected.

- Professional integrity: This means having the capacity and motivation to take responsibility and accept challenges, to admit and learn from mistakes and to demonstrate respect and equality of care for all. Patients' needs will be put before one's own when appropriate.

Below are examples of typical questions in these three areas. The examples also demonstrate the two main question formats:

- Where rank ordering is required a correct order has been decided by consensus. Full marks will be obtained when the choices are put in the correct order. A small variation such as reversing the first and second options will only result in a small reduction in marks. A zero mark is only given when the whole order is reversed by a candidate.

- Where a candidate has to choose possible correct options from a list then a mark is awarded for each correct item chosen.

Example 1

Question   You are a foundation doctor working on a busy surgical unit. On theatre days you often find you have to deal with difficult ward problems without adequate supervision from senior colleagues. You are unhappy about this.

Rank the possible responses below in the most suitable order.

1   Discuss the situation with your consultant

2   Discuss the situation with your foundation programme director

3   Seek advice from experienced nurses on the unit when in difficulty

4   Seek advice from other foundation colleagues when you have difficulty

Answer   1 2 4 3

This question deals with coping with pressure and, in particular, recognising limitations and establishing effective strategies. Foundation doctors should always have easy access to senior cover. The person most likely to be able to sort things out is your consultant and failing that your programme director who should have influence over the way foundation doctors are trained in the hospital. Both the other options are inappropriate but asking doctors is slightly better than asking nurses because of the nature of their training.

Example 2

Question You are in a general practice surgery. A 40-year-old man whom you referred to hospital with abdominal pain was found to have multiple liver and peritoneal metastases from an earlier colonic carcinoma. The local oncologist thinks he is unsuitable for chemotherapy and is now terminally ill. He has been advised by a family member who is a nurse at a regional oncology centre to see a specialist there who does clinical trials and he asks if you can refer him.

Rank the possible responses below in the most suitable order.

1 Advise him that this is not a suitable option

2 Discuss with him his feelings and expectations about a possible referral

3 Speak to the local oncologist about the request

4 Speak to the regional specialist about the request

Answer 2 3 4 1

This question deals with empathy and sensitivity and in particular responding to the needs and concerns of the patient. None of these options are wrong and indeed it is unlikely that chemotherapy will help him. However, the main issue here is to find out what the patient is thinking and what he feels his needs are. As he has asked for a referral this is most likely what he wants. Professional etiquette dictates that you talk to the local oncologist first. He may be able to advise you and perhaps even make the referral himself.

Example 3

Question You are in a general practice surgery. A 50-year-old man has a red scaly lesion behind one ear. Two years earlier a local dermatologist was quite definite about a diagnosis of seborrhoeic eczema and he prescribed a moderately potent steroid cream. The patient does not think the cream was effective when he used it 2 years ago. He has had no treatment since and has come back to see you in the GP surgery because the lesion is still present. There is a small area of ulceration in the centre and you are concerned he may be developing a squamous cell carcinoma.

Select from the list below the three most suitable responses at this consultation.

1 Arrange a biopsy to be carried out in the practice

2 Ask your supervisor to come in and have a look at the lesion

3 Offer to review him in one month to see if there is any worsening of the lesion

4 Prescribe a more potent steroid

5 Prescribe the same steroid that he had 2 years ago

6 Refer him back to the original consultant

7 Refer him to a different consultant

Answer   1 2 6

This question is in the area of professional integrity and in particular a willingness to back one's own professional judgement. Here you are told that you suspect the lesion is a squamous cell carcinoma. This means that you think the consultant made an incorrect diagnosis and presumably the diagnosis should have been that of a precancerous lesion such as actinic keratosis or Bowen disease. It is hard for a junior doctor to contradict a senior colleague. If there is an easily available second opinion such as the clinical supervisor then it is obvious that this should be the first course of action. If you are correct then the patient needs an urgent biopsy either in hospital or the practice. The original consultant should have the opportunity to know about and learn from his mistake and a referral to another consultant would only be appropriate if the patient expressed a preference for this. None of the other options are appropriate.

The personal skills that are being tested in Stage 2 should have been acquired during undergraduate and foundation training so no special preparation should be necessary apart from becoming familiar with the format of the test. It is useful to discuss with educational supervisors. The wider issues involved in the complex medical and management problems encountered in everyday practice. Also, regular case analysis and discussion with colleagues is a good way to practice and develop competences in this area.

The necessary attributes of a doctor are defined by the General Medical Council and can be accessed via their website[5] or through their various publications, particularly *Good Medical Practice*[6]

REFERENCES

4   The National Recruitment Office for General Practice Training website (www.gprecruitment.org.uk).

5   General Medical Council. Good Medical Practice (2006). Available at: www.gmc-uk.org/guidance/good_medical_practice

6   General Medical Council. *Good Medical Practice*. London: General Medical Council, 2006.References 2 and 3 seem to be the same, ie Good Medical Practice 2006. Is the information on the website different from that in the publication?

Chapter 14
Professional
Dilemmas

QUESTIONS

14.1   You are a foundation doctor in accident and emergency. A
40-year-old man complains of a flu-like illness for 1 week
with cough but no shortness of breath. He is apyrexial
and has a clear chest. The patient informs you that he is a
consultant anaesthetist from Australia on holiday in the UK.
He demands antibiotics, specifically an expensive new one
which is rarely used in the UK but 'we use it all the time back
home for chest infections'.

Rank the possible responses below in the most suitable
order.

1   Advise him that it good practice not to prescribe antibiotics
immediately for a flu-like illness, that he should take symptomatic
relief and consult a doctor again if things get worse or do not
improve in a reasonable amount of time

2   Ask for advice from your consultant/registrar on the shop floor

3   Politely ask him if he can give evidence of his professional
qualifications before prescribing

4   Respect his expectation and prescribe the requested antibiotic

14.2   You are a foundation doctor in psychiatry. You cover a busy
acute psychiatric ward, divided into two groups, each under
a different consultant. You gradually realise that the other
trainee cannot cope with her work. She frequently hides in
the doctor's office, does not complete the tasks requested
by the nurses, and rarely reviews her patients by herself.
However, she takes good notes from ward rounds and
her consultant does not seem to have any issues with her

work. No-one else has yet commented on this. You can only just manage the workload from the patients under your consultant.

Rank the possible responses below in the most suitable order.

1 Cover your colleague's work

2 Discuss the problem with her consultant

3 Report her to hospital management

4 Raise the issue directly with your colleague

14.3 Nursing staff tell you the 19-year-old son of one of your patients is waiting to talk with you about his mother's condition. She has just been told she has breast cancer and is about to undergo further investigations to determine the management.

Rank the possible responses below in the most suitable order.

1 Offer to discuss things with his mother present

2 Read the patient's notes, and take them in with you to fully provide any information the son needs about his mother

3 See the son, listen to his concerns and explain about any procedures he is worried about without revealing any confidential information

4 Tell the nursing staff to tell the son to discuss it with his mother

14.4 You are a foundation doctor based in a busy GP surgery for 4 months. Unfortunately all the consulting rooms are occupied and you can only see patients in surgery between the hours of 11:30 and 14:00.

Rank the possible responses below in the most suitable order.

1   Discuss with the practice manager to try to identify possible slots in which you can reschedule some of your surgeries

2   It is better not to complain and accept the situation

3   Report the practice to the foundation programme director

4   Use the rest of the time to sit in with other team members or seek alternative activities in the practice

14.5   During the final week of your foundation attachment in general practice a patient you have been looking after gives you a thank you card. Inside, you find a cheque for £200.

Rank the possible responses below in the most suitable order.

1   Happily accept the gift as a just reward for your efforts

2   Identify your feeling of embarrassment at receiving the gift and refuse

3   Offer to use the money to buy some equipment for the surgery

4   Politely talk to the patient to ascertain the reason for the gift

14.6   You suspect that a colleague in your hospital firm is misusing alcohol. He seems sober when at work but at mess parties and when out socially you have noticed that he usually gets quite drunk.

Rank the possible responses below in the most suitable order.

1   Discuss matters with him directly as you know him well

2   Discuss matters with other colleagues to get their views

3   Discuss matters with your consultant or the firm's clinical director

4   Report him to the General Medical Council (GMC)

14.7   You are working in accident and emergency. A 30-year-old woman complains of shortness of breath, chest pain and shaking hands. She does not smoke and has no family history of note. She also complains of tingling around her mouth. Her observations are normal blood pressure, pulse of 100 and respiratory rate of 15–18 (variable). An electrocardiogram (ECG) is normal, and examination is normal apart from these observations. She is very anxious. You diagnose a panic attack and reassure her that the problem is not heart or lung related, and discharge her. After she is gone your registrar, who had not seen the patient, reviews the case and says that with a tachycardia and shortness of breath we should exclude a pulmonary embolism and she should have had a D-dimer test. He recommends you call her back in for this.

Rank the possible responses below in the most suitable order.

1   Arrange for the patient to be called back immediately for the test

2   Discuss with the registrar that your clinical judgement was that she did not have a serious physical illness and that you did take a proper history and examine her

3   Learn from this and consider doing more investigations in future before discharging a patient

4   Telephone the patient, see how she is feeling, and depending on the outcome you may offer investigations

14.8   You are a foundation doctor on rotation in general practice. During a consultation, a patient complains about the attitude of one of the reception staff. What do you do?

Rank the possible responses below in the most suitable order.

1   Address the complaint with the member of staff directly

2 Outline the practice's complaints procedure and ask the patient to speak to the practice manager

3 Try to calm the patient's concerns and stop this complaint becoming more serious

4 Raise the incident at the next partners' meeting

14.9   **In your work as a foundation doctor in general practice you find one of the receptionists having a look at the medical records of a patient you have seen that morning. The patient and her family are well known to the practice as frequent consulters and live in the house next door.**

Rank the possible responses below in the most suitable order.

1 Address your concerns about records at the practice meeting

2 Discuss the matter with your trainer

3 Informally ask the receptionist what she is doing

4 Report the matter to the practice manager

14.10   **One of the patients under your care as a foundation year 2 doctor remains unconscious following a stroke. A colleague, who practises acupuncture, says she would like to see whether this is helpful in helping the patient regain consciousness. What do you do?**

Rank the possible responses below in the most suitable order.

1 Discuss the idea with the your senior colleagues and consultant

2 Dismiss this notion as ridiculous

3 Involve the patient's family in any decision making

4 Seek advice from the hospital authorities and your defence organisation

14.11   You are in general practice visiting an 86-year-old man with moderately severe chronic obstructive pulmonary disease, complaining of worsening shortness of breath. He frequently calls out general practitioners and is occasionally admitted to hospital for a few days. The respiratory nurse specialists visit him fortnightly to avoid unnecessary admissions, and had sent a note to the practice the previous day saying that he was very anxious but they did not consider admission necessary. On examination his pulse is 100 and regular and he is tachypnoeic. His oxygen saturation is 94% on air, which is normal for him. On auscultating his chest, there are widespread coarse crackles. He says that he will not cope at home tonight and begs to be admitted to hospital. He admits to being lonely and prefers the hospital as he receives more attention.

Rank the possible responses below in the most suitable order.

1   Admit him to hospital

2   Advise him that he is no worse than usual and that you will not admit him

3   Discuss with the patient benefits of admission versus staying at home

4   Telephone the hospital 'rapid response' admission avoidance team

14.12   You are in general practice and your surgery is running half an hour late. Your patient is a 35-year-old woman with chronic back pain and sciatica who takes regular paracetamol, tramadol and gabapentin. She also has moderate depression with occasional severe exacerbations and takes citalopram. She has a history of repeated deliberate self-harm. The patient asks for a repeat prescription of all her pain medications, as the last supply issued 1 week ago has gone missing from her flat. You notice before she comes in that in the previous consultation last week she was referred to the acute mental health home treatment team because of suicidal thoughts following a recent relationship breakdown. When you mention this, she assures you that she no longer feels suicidal and is taking her citalopram regularly. She says it is mainly the pain that is getting her down.

Rank the possible responses below in the most suitable order.

1   Ask her to wait in the waiting room and phone the home treatment team and ask for their opinion on her mental state and suicide risk, and find out their plans

2   Examine her mental state further before prescribing

3   Issue her with a week's supply of medication

4   Issue the prescription and plan to telephone the home treatment team after surgery

14.13   As a foundation doctor in general practice you notice some old and new bruises on the legs of a woman who you often see with minor illnesses. You suspect domestic violence. What do you do?

Rank the possible responses below in the most suitable order.

1   Call social services and ask for a domestic assessment

2   Contact her partner, also a patient of yours, and ask him what he has been doing to her

3   Ignore the bruises and hope that she will ask for help when she feels ready

4   Raise the issue by asking her how she sustained the bruises

14.14 It is the weekend and the plastic surgery ward staff asks you to prescribe analgesia for one of their postoperative patients. When you go to see the patient it is clear they find you attractive, and they tell you they have just ended a long-term relationship and are looking for a fresh start. The patient says they will be discharged the following day, and asks you out on a date the following weekend.

Rank the possible responses below in the most suitable order.

1 Discuss the matter with colleagues

2 Gently explain that your duties of a doctor preclude any relationship

3 Report them to the hospital management for sexual harassment

4 Wait until they are discharged before accepting

14.15 You are a foundation doctor coming to the end of a busy surgical job, and your colleague working on the same ward contracts chickenpox. He may be absent for up to 4 weeks. You usually cover the ward for each other to attend clinic twice per week and to assist in theatre whenever possible. You do not think you will be able to cope with all the work alone.

Rank the possible responses below in the most suitable order.

1 Arrange cover with other colleagues

2 Complain to hospital management of overwork

3 Discuss your workload with your consultant

4 Make sure outpatients is informed that you may be called away

14.16 You are a foundation doctor in general surgery. Your child's nursery (on the hospital site) telephones to say that your 1-year-old has a temperature of 38°C and needs to be picked up as soon as possible. Your partner is 50 miles away on business and you are due to assist your consultant in theatre.

Rank the possible responses below in the most suitable order.

1 Apologise to your consultant and go to pick up your daughter. He can arrange another assistant

2 Arrange for a colleague to cover in return for you helping them out later

3 Explain your situation to the nursery. You pay them to look after your child so they can keep her until the end of the day

4 Phone around friends to find someone else to pick up your daughter

14.17 You are working in a busy city practice. You realise that the next patient on your list is a teacher at your son's primary school. She obviously does not know it is you she is due to see. The appointment screen says the problem is 'personal'.

Rank the possible responses below in the most suitable order.

1 Arrange for another doctor to see the patient, explaining why to both him and the patient

2 Ask the patient whether she would like to still see you, or another doctor

3 See the patient, reassuring her very carefully that you are impeccably confidential

4 You should make sure that everyone you know is aware of where you work to avoid this happening

14.18 You are a foundation year 2 trainee working in accident and emergency. During one of your regular training sessions with the other junior doctors the consultant highlights the missed fractures that have been detected via routine radiology review. You recognise that one of these is a patient you saw and realise you are one of the doctors who missed a fracture. What should you do?

Choose the three most appropriate options from the list below.

1 Amend the patient's notes highlighting why this was a difficult X-ray to interpret

2 Ask for senior review of X-rays before discharging patients

3 Listen carefully to the training to see if there is anything that can improve your skills

4 Speak to the consultant to see if there are any specific learning points to be aware of

5 Stop reviewing X-rays

6 Write to the patient apologising for the mistake

14.19 You are a doctor in accident and emergency. A colleague on the same rota has just been accepted on to a course he really wants to attend and asks you to cover his night shift next Wednesday. You will be working 08:00 to 18:00 all week and this means you would not have enough time to get home between shifts. He offers to pay you the standard locum rate. You will be working together for the next few months and you do not want to offend him.

Choose the three most appropriate options from the list below.

1 Advise your colleague to discuss the issue with his consultant and offer to rearrange your sessions to help if needed

2 Do the night shift but call in sick the next day as it will be easier to find locum cover in the daytime

3   Do the shift plus your own work and rely on short naps during quiet periods to combat fatigue

4   Discuss the problem with other colleagues to formulate a solution

5   Discuss with your consultant and offer to work the night shift if the day shifts can be covered to allow you enough rest

6   Refuse to cover him because he should have been more organised with his study leave request

14.20   You are in General Practice doing telephone triage. You speak to a patient who seems anxious and says she is 'very unwell'. She has severe sleep problems due to restless legs syndrome secondary to chronic renal failure and is due a follow up appointment at the local sleep clinic in 6 weeks' time. She has previously asked one of the partners to fax the clinic and bring the appointment forward as she is not sleeping at all. There is no mention of this in your colleague's notes, just discussion of her other medical problems. She has discontinued the medication recommended by the clinic as it was 'no use'. She becomes verbally aggressive when you try to take a more detailed history and demands you promise to send the fax straightaway.

Choose the three most appropriate options from the list below.

1   Ask her if she would mind being more polite over the telephone. Agree to write to the clinic requesting they see her sooner

2   Assure the patient you do have her interests to heart and will fax the sleep clinic straightaway

3   Discuss her anxiety and offer a further appointment in the surgery to think further about other options while waiting for the clinic appointment

4   Discuss her expectations of referral times to a non-emergency clinic and advise her to reconsider in the meantime trying the medication they recommend

5   Say you will wait until tomorrow and discuss the issue with your colleague who is not in surgery today

6   Suggest that this is not an emergency and the sleep clinic is following her up at an appropriate interval

14.21   You are working in general practice and discover an abnormal smear result (severe dyskaryosis), which has not been acted on. The result was sent to your practice 6 months ago. The practice nurse tells you that this has happened before. What steps would you take next?

Choose the three most appropriate options from the list below.

1   Ask the nurse to do a further smear today

2   Contact your medical defence society for advice

3   Discuss the issue at a practice significant event meeting

4   Send an urgent referral for colposcopy

5   Telephone the patient to come in and discuss the matter

6   Write to the patient outlining what has happened and inviting her to come and discuss the matter if she wishes

ANSWERS

14.1   **1 2 4 3**

This question focuses on balancing local evidence-based guidelines, patient choice and the problems faced when dealing with colleagues whose views may differ from our own. It is in the area of professional integrity and backing your own judgement. It is irrelevant whether this man is a real doctor, but having said that, if he is, it will be diplomatically challenging to differ from his opinion being his junior. Asking for his qualifications may just prove difficult and not help matters. We are told to respect patients' ideas, concerns and expectations but not at the expense of practising good medicine. It is always useful to ask a colleague for advice.

14.2   **4 2 3 1**

This question is about professional integrity, sensitivity to colleagues and concern for patients' welfare. It may be that you can help her with support and advice and if not you her consultant may be best placed. However, if she is underperforming we have a duty to 'whistle blow' and management will need informing. Covering for her may overburden you and endanger patient safety.

14.3   **3 1 2 4**

This is another question about professional integrity and respect for patient confidentiality. Relatives do often ask to speak with doctors about their own concerns. Often these relate to the technical aspects of management, as the terms used can be confusing and worrying for people with no medical background. Allowing them time and space to air their concerns is often enough, and reassures them that you will care for their loved one. If there are any specific questions relating to the patient, or prognosis, you need to be careful not to disclose any confidential information. Gently explaining that you have a duty to keep this information confidential, but are happy to listen to any information they feel would be important for you to know, will often be satisfactory. When a patient indicates they would like you to share certain information with their relatives, it may be appropriate to discuss this with them in the presence of the patient. However, use caution when answering patient's questions in front of others, as the patient may not know where the answers will lead.

14.4   1 4 3 2

This question is in the area of coping with pressure, finding strategies to cope and not losing sight of the wider picture. Due to recent changes in medical education, there are many more doctors rotating through general practice than ever before and places need to be found for everyone. This means it may be difficult to provide dedicated accommodation for foundation doctors, and the team may not all be familiar with this role. It is important early on to establish with your trainer what your objectives are from this training. Sitting in on surgeries with your trainer and other doctors is an important element, as is learning more about the other members of the primary healthcare team. However, you will be expected to see patients in your own surgeries, even if occasionally at unusual times. If access to your own surgeries is a consistent problem it may be best to discuss this with the practice manager, who may be able to reorganise other activities in the practice to allow this. The practice manager can let you know when consulting rooms are free when staff are away. It is unreasonable to have to put up with this every day so if no attempt is made to introduce more flexibility the programme director would need to review the suitability of the practice for training.

14.5   4 3 2 1

This question is in the area of professional integrity and empathy/ sensitivity. The patient may genuinely wish to reward you so it is easy to offend if the gift is quickly rebuffed. However it may be best to explore sensitively for less appropriate motives or if the patient can really afford the gift. It would be inappropriate to accept the gift on one's own behalf. Many practices do have policies (eg buying equipment, patient fund) for dealing with gifts and those over £100 should be registered (Health and Social Care Bill, 2000). Doctors will vary in their reaction to such a gift but as long as the practice policy is not one of outright refusal then the ranking above seems reasonable.

14.6   1 2 3 4

This question is in the area of empathy/sensitivity, responding to the needs of a colleague but also professional integrity, looking at the risks for patients. This question is tricky and there is more than one approach. Depending on your relationship with the colleague, you can speak to them directly, though this may be difficult or intimidating, especially if he is a senior colleague. Discussing it among your other colleagues first helps to encourage ownership of an important issue and aids the gathering of views and information. If you find that your concerns are well founded, your consultant needs to be involved and ultimately the GMC. Alcoholism calls fitness to practise into question. Your colleague should be supported medically although you should not be medically involved in treating him.

14.7   4 2 3 1

This question deals with the concepts of sensitivity and professional integrity. You made a clinical judgement which has now been questioned – how should you react? A senior colleague has told you that you have omitted a test he would see as essential; it would look negligent to ignore this. You need to consider whether you really did miss a test out and be open to learning from these situations, or you might have been right. It certainly warrants further discussion with the registrar especially if you are confident in your decision. The patient may have some views on this and may have improved or deteriorated depending on her physical pathology or emotional state. She may be reassured or worried by the test, and she may be made more anxious by coming in. It is fair to discuss it with her, but you must do so sensitively, taking into account her ideas, concerns and expectations.

14.8   3 2 4 1

This question raises issues of empathy and sensitivity, and dealing with a potentially stressful situation. We must realise that many processes may have taken place before any encounter between doctor and patient in the consulting room. Patients may have had an unfavourable experience with a member of staff, but we must act in a non-judgemental way and not take sides. It is important to empathise with the patient, and this could just be a way for them to 'let off steam', and they may not wish to take things further. However, in some instances, people may wish to make a formal, written complaint and so they should be aware of the procedure. If the issue is to be raised with the staff member then a senior member of the practice should do so.

14.9   3 2 4 1

This question is in the area of professional integrity. Patient records are confidential and should only be accessed by relevant staff for relevant reasons. There may be a plausible explanation in this case, but if there is not then this needs to be addressed. There may be other aspects of inappropriate behaviour or breaches of privacy in the practice, and this needs to be dealt with from a senior level. Your trainer should be able to provide guidance on how best to deal with this.

14.10   1 4 3 2

This is a novel situation and unlikely to be encountered in day to day practice but it raises issues regarding efficacy of treatments and what is allowed to be practised within the National Health Service. Certainly in some surgeries, trained acupuncturists see patients and can help in many conditions. Usually, these are musculoskeletal problems. In the hospital setting, there may be several barriers to this type of treatment. It would need to be discussed at a higher level and with relevant advice from your defence society and possibly the hospital ethics committee. The question is about empathy and sensitivity and acting in an open and non-judgemental manner.

14.11   3 4 1 2

This is about coping under pressure as well as empathy/sensitivity. The opinion of other professionals needs to be taken into account – but remember that you have seen the patient more recently and the others are specifically seeking to avoid admission. The patient's views are also important but if admission is really unnecessary clinically, then you should not be persuaded by him. You should be sensitive to this man's home circumstances. If he is agreeable 'rapid response' may be able to provide adequate short-term domiciliary support.

14.12   2 1 3 4

The fear here is that this woman may be storing medication for a suicide attempt. The doctor is under pressure because of this and the time pressures. Some people lead chaotic lives so it is possible the tablets have gone missing or been mislaid. Empathy and sensitivity are important. The doctor should stay calm. It is their decision whether to prescribe so a proper assessment of suicide risk can be made and if it is felt to be low a prescription can be issued. This is professional integrity and backing one's own judgement. Given the circumstances it is important to liaise with colleagues and issue only a small amount of medication. Doctors can be too trusting, so to issue the full prescription before knowing the whole story may be foolish.

14.13   4 3 1 2

This is a difficult scenario but it is important to address the cause of the bruises, otherwise you could be seen to be colluding with the perpetrator. Addressing this sensitively when the woman is present in the room on her own is important rather than in front of any third party, who could also be involved. If she is not ready to tell you, you must realise that she may be fearful or guilty or anxious, so it is important to build trust so that she can seek help from you when appropriate. You would like to have her permission before involving an outside agency, but this may not always be forthcoming and you will want to act in her best interest as you see it. The question tests empathy and sensitivity responding to and understanding the woman's needs and concerns while at the same time maintaining an appropriate distance and not becoming over sensitive as if personally involved.

14.14   2 1 3 4

This question is about professional integrity. The General Medical Council has recently updated its guidance in *Duties of a Doctor*. Here it states that 'You must not use your professional position to establish or pursue a sexual or improper emotional relationship with a patient or someone close to them'. This is generally taken to mean that relationships with patients or their relatives are considered inappropriate, even if the patient has been discharged from your care, if you met through your professional work. This is partly due to the special nature of the doctor–patient relationship, which means patients or relatives often confide intimate and private thoughts and feelings at times of great stress, and may not feel the same once things settle. In the above situation, the patient's judgement may be impaired by several factors, including the anaesthetic, social isolation, unfamiliar surroundings, frightening clinical procedures and by the pain that they are experiencing. For these reasons they may feel attraction to someone in a position of caring for them. They need to trust that the doctor will not misuse this position. In general as the doctor it is your responsibility to understand the reasons behind the request for a date, and treat the matter sensitively and professionally. However, if you feel intimidated by advances made by a patient it is a good idea to discuss your feelings with a trusted senior colleague.

14.15   3 4 1 2

In the first instance you should discuss your workload with the consultant, as they will be aware of the sickness absence and may already have considered alternatives. It will be helpful if you can present them with ideas for a solution to the problem. As a junior member of the team you should be supernumerary and not relied on. However, in practice it is difficult for the team to provide sufficient training opportunities on a regular basis without starting to depend on the presence of the junior. It is a good idea to make sure the outpatient department is aware of the situation, as sufficient patients will have been booked to provide you with training, which means that in your absence the clinic is likely to over-run and they need to explain this to patients. Also, it will help them to manage the bookings and cancellations for the next few weeks. If you merely cover the ward for the next few weeks you may miss valuable theatre training opportunities. Personally asking colleagues to cover your bleep would be one option. However, everyone is busy and any contingencies for cover should be ratified by the consultant, as they may have had other plans for reorganising the team during this period.

14.16   4 2 1 3

This question is mainly about planning ahead to ensure that work and family life are compatible. If you are to survive being a successful doctor with young children (at any stage of your career) you need to have contingency plans to cope with this sort of pressure. You may not be able to immediately drop everything to pick up your child from nursery. Colleagues and friends may be able to help and you need to be prepared to ask, and offer help in return. Other systems may not be ideal (such as the ability of a nursery to care for a sick child, or sick leave rules), but you will just have to work around them.

14.17   2 1 3 4

This is an embarrassing situation potentially for doctor and patient but will inevitably happen occasionally. It is not practical to make sure everyone knows where you work. In deciding the best options you need to think about the principles of autonomy, beneficence and non-maleficence. Autonomy usually wins but your patient must not come to harm. Only they will know if seeing a doctor they know in another situation will affect their view of the care received. Obviously you will act professionally and uphold confidentiality and should ensure they are clear about this. You should not treat family or friends as there is a risk of making emotionally involved decisions.

14.18   2 3 4

As a junior member of the team in a training role, it is assumed that you will have access to senior colleagues for difficult situations such as interpreting X-rays. There is a learning curve for all grades of junior doctor, and the fail-safe mechanism of formal radiology reporting is in place to detect fractures that are subtle and otherwise may be missed. If the patient were to complain in such a case, it would be the responsibility of the consultant to respond, although you may be asked for your input when they are drafting this response. It is also their responsibility to determine the action taken with juniors under these circumstances, and it may be that in this case all the juniors would benefit from additional radiology training. It is clearly wrong to amend patient case notes after the event. Being able to admit mistakes and learn from them is part of professional integrity.

14.19   1 4 5

Accident and emergency is a busy job with the need for 24-hour cover. It is difficult to find locum cover at short notice and doctors are advised to give as much notice as possible of leave requests. However, there will be times when colleagues ask favours at short notice, and there is the need to be flexible, without compromising your ability to function safely. To simply refuse may lead to a difficult working relationship, particularly in accident and emergency where staff need to pull together as a team. Discussing the matter with your colleague's consultant may make him reassess the importance of this course or the consultant may take steps to provide cover. Allowing your consultant the chance to suggest a solution and offering flexibility in your shifts is one option, but working together as a team to swap shifts and find a solution that suits everyone would also be good. This solution would obviously need ratification and when changing rotas care should be taken to ensure people are clear about when they are expected to be in the department. The question is mainly in the area of empathy and sensitivity, responding to the needs of others with understanding.

14.20   2 3 4

This question tests coping with pressure. This woman is behaving unacceptably but does have a chronic illness and may have problems that you are unable to pick up over the telephone. It would be inappropriate to address her behaviour directly as it may make her worse and risk complaints. It is worth trying to explore why she is behaving like this and not attempting to put her down. However, she needs to be given realistic expectations.

14.21   1 4 5

This situation needs addressing promptly, and you need to take personal responsibility for this issue, rather than hoping the patient may respond to your letter. With a telephone call you know the patient has received your message. You need to be open and honest about the delay as it may have a bearing on clinical outcome. Non-disclosure is only justified if you think it will adversely affect the patient's mental well-being. Obviously, you should also explain what severe dyskaryosis is. It is important that this incident is looked into further, to ensure it does not happen again. Therefore discussion at a practice significant event meeting openly and honestly is part of the learning from this incident. You may also choose to write to the patient to outline what processes have been remedied to avoid a repeat of the incident (e.g. designated clinician receiving all smear results and correlating them with a logbook of smears taken to avoid omissions). The question tests professional integrity.

INDEX

Locators refer to question number.